MASTER LAM'S
WALKING
CHI KUNG

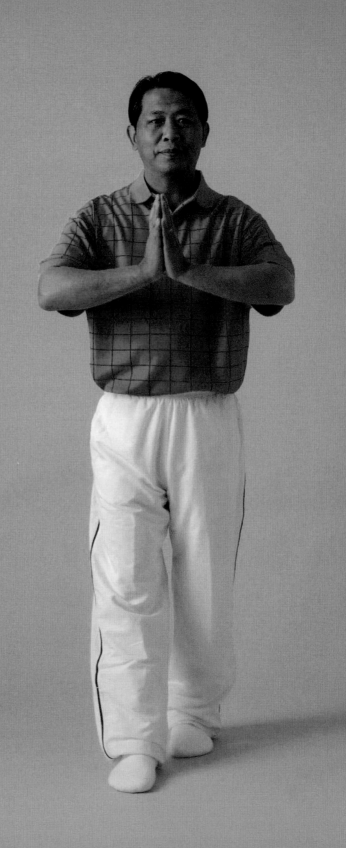

MASTER LAM'S
WALKING CHI KUNG

Master Lam Kamchuen

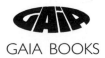

GAIA BOOKS

A GAIA ORIGINAL

Books from Gaia celebrate the vision of Gaia, the self-sustaining living Earth, and seek to help its readers live in greater personal and planetary harmony.

Editor Cindy Engel

Project Editor Camilla Davis

Designer Bridget Morley

Photography Paul Forrester

Production Louise Hall

Direction Jo Godfrey Wood, Patrick Nugent

® This is a Registered Trade Mark of Gaia Books

First published in the United Kingdom in 2006
by Gaia Books, a division of Octopus Publishing Group Ltd
2–4 Heron Quays, London E14 4JP

Distributed in the United States and Canada by
Sterling Publishing Co., Inc.
387 Park Avenue South, New York, NY 10016–8810

ISBN-13: 978-1-85675-235-0
ISBN-10: 1-85675-235-6

A CIP catalogue record of this book is available from the British Library.

Printed and bound in China

10 9 8 7 6 5 4 3 2 1

CAUTION
The techniques, ideas, and suggestions in this book are to be used at the reader's sole discretion and risk. Always follow the instructions carefully, observe the cautions, and consult a doctor about any medical conditions.

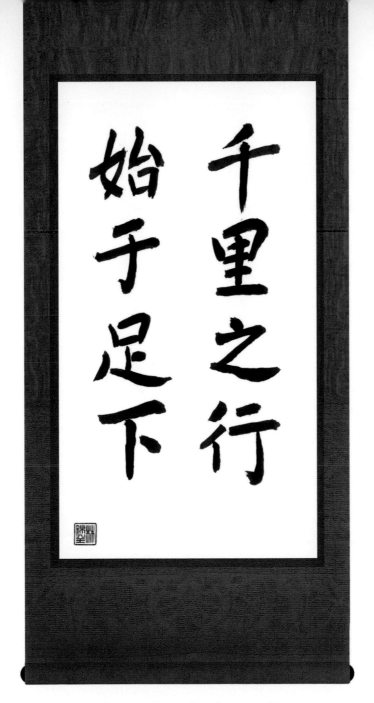

The journey of a thousand li
begins from beneath the legs.

(A 'li' is a Chinese unit of measure equal to 576 m [630 yd].)

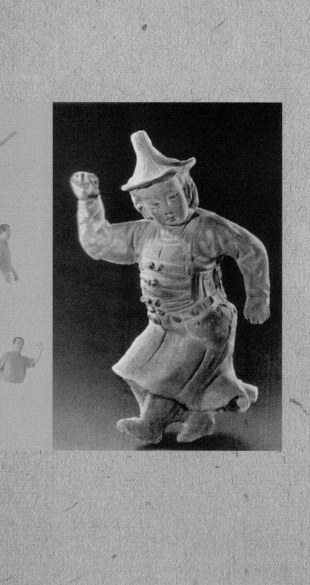

CONTENTS

Origins of Walking Chi Kung

*In order to do anything in this life,
we must first have energy.*

GUAN TSE, ANCIENT CHINESE PHILOSOPHER

The marvels of modern technology and science have transformed our way of life. However, our modern lives are characterized by daily hubbubs and demanding schedules. Anxiety and tension have become the norm in our everyday routine. Somehow, despite all our modern marvels, we live in a more stressful world than our forefathers'.

Peace and quiet have become elusive. Increasingly, people are recognizing this and turning their attention to the East, where greater emphasis is often given to leading a harmonious lifestyle. The ancient Chinese arts are being rediscovered by the Western world and becoming part of a global culture.

The Chinese understand all human actions (whether mental, physical, or spiritual) to be manifestations of the dynamics of an individual's energy.

With this understanding, each human body is seen to be a reservoir of energies. The body is but flesh-deep; an external structure housing something greater. It is like a great lake, not merely defined by its shoreline. Each human life is governed by the dynamics of the body's energy.

For countless years, the ancient Chinese painstakingly observed and studied this dynamism. Undaunted, they looked not only at the human body but also at the universe. The reward for their efforts was the discovery and understanding of Chi. The concept of Chi became a pillar of Eastern philosophy.

ELUSIVE CHI

Chi is the primal medium of which all things in this universe are made. It is the energy, or life force, which forms the essence of everything. Current understanding of this elusive, intangible Chi, results from the collective efforts of hundreds of Chinese scholars over a few thousand years. To understand Chi is to have an appreciation of universal energy.

The concept of Chi is applied far and wide. In China, it is used and needed in medicine, geography, Feng Shui (Chinese placement geometry), climatology, even in cookery. This book focuses on the working of Chi within the body.

The Chinese choice of the term Chi is a story all of its own. The contemporary, officially accepted, character denotes 'breath' or 'air'. It is because of this translation that Chi Kung is often mistaken as the practice of simple breathing exercises, yet this choice of character is worthy of consideration, for Chi is formless and insubstantial like air. Sometimes, Chi is translated as 'aura', but this is still a derivative of the word, air.

The ancient Chinese character for Chi conveys a different meaning that reflects a deeper understanding. It is portrayed by two elements interacting one upon the other. The whole character embodies the concept of a furnace as being representative of Chi (see right, and pages 24–25).

Chi is the true face of the inner strength of all things. When you look at a great old tree, it radiates immeasurable strength and power. The exterior is neither threatening nor dangerous, yet somehow you are intimidated and dwarfed by its presence.

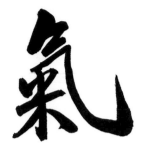

Above *The contemporary character for Chi denotes 'breath' or 'air'.* **On the right** *is the calligraphy for 'flow of chi'. The lower character is the ancient Chinese character for Chi. It comprises two elements that, when viewed together, embody the concept of a furnace. The element at the top represents a pot or cauldron with two legs and possibly a handle. The element below represents leaping flames, heating the cauldron.*

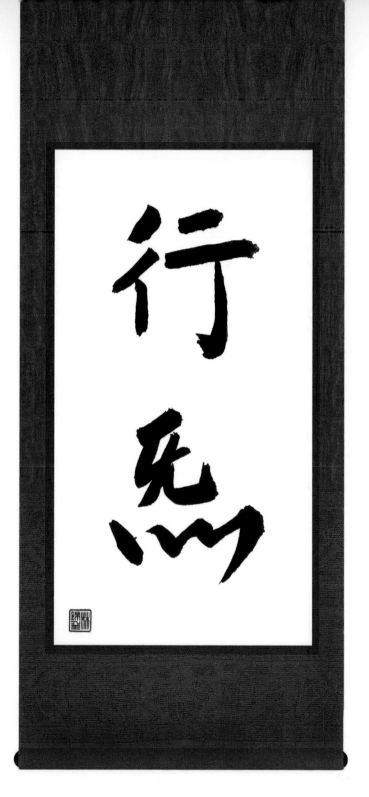

Chi Kung

The manifestation of Chi is everywhere, including the human body. The Chinese study of human energy can be traced back to the reign of the Yellow Emperor, thought to be around 2690–2590 BC. Despite its age, the study of Chi remains an active field of study, and continues to be researched in China and other parts of the world.

Properly harnessed, energy can be brought to new highs and greater intensity. A human, being a field of energy, can also be brought to a higher level – physically, mentally, and spiritually – given appropriate cultivation.

One of the greatest legacies of Chinese civilization is the cultivation of human energy. The name, Chi Kung, literally translates as 'the working of Chi'. It is an internal energy practice that stimulates the flow of Chi throughout the human body.

Chi Kung works the channels through which human energy flows, and harmonizes the life force so that the person achieves a natural balance. Chi Kung is, therefore, a process of change and transformation that improves mental and physical health.

The practice of Chi Kung is varied – ranging from static standing postures, sitting and laying down, to the emulation of animal movements found in nature. Hence, there are various schools and styles, each with its own emphasis on health, spiritual improvement, or martial development.

Chi Kung is applied in many different fields and areas of expertise, satisfying various needs. Though the techniques and aims may differ in detail, the underlying philosophy is the same for all of them.

ORIGINS

Like many great arts, Chi Kung does not originate from a single source. It is not like holding a thread in a maze, follow it and eventually you will get out. If you tried to do that, you would find yourself trapped in a cobweb of threads.

The art of Chi Kung is like a river formed from numerous tributaries into one unified force. As you move upstream, you find that the river has multiple sources.

There are four principle origins of Chi Kung. This ancient art can be traced back to the monasteries of the Buddhist faith, the schools of Taoist academics, the practices of herbalists and doctors, and the disciplines of martial artists.

THE LINEAGE

With virtually no external movements, Zhan Zhuang (pronounced Jam Jong) is the most potent form of Chi Kung developed. It is a unique exercise system concentrating entirely on the inner workings of the human body through a variety of carefully composed postures. Zhan Zhuang means 'Standing Like a Tree' and reference to this practice can be traced back as far as Lao Tse's writings in the *Tao Te Ching*. The practice does as it suggests: it develops great inner strength like that of a magnificent mature tree.

Zhan Zhuang, in turn, is part of a greater body of training. It is the foundation of many different disciplines of martial arts. It is also the underlying element of the martial art, Da Cheng Chuan, 'The Great Accomplishment', founded by Grand Master Wang Xiang Zhai. Through his discoveries and teachings,

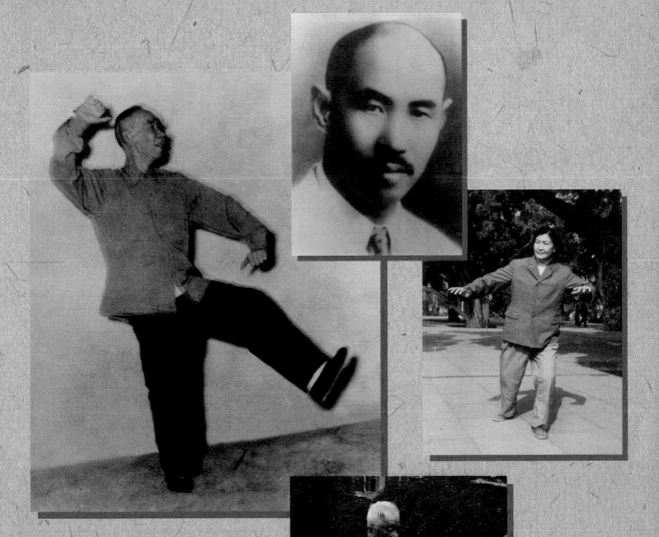

Top An early portrait of a young Wang Xiang Zhai.
Centre right Madame Wang, the daughter of Grand Master Wang, practises in a Beijing park.
Bottom Professor Yu, a student of Grand Master Wang and in turn the teacher of Master Lam, maintains the lineage in China.
Centre left Grand Master Wang during practice.

he has indirectly helped millions of people to greater health. One of his disciples, Professor Yu Yong Nian, initially practised dentistry but, intrigued by the health benefits of this art, studied under Grand Master Wang Xiang Zhai and eventually became a leading authority on Chi Kung. As his disciple, I am now honoured to pass on the teachings of this tradition.

LITERATURE ON LEGS

*The journey of a thousand li
    begins from beneath the legs.*

Grand Master Wang Xiang Zhai, Professor Yu, and I, have placed unparalleled importance on working the lower limbs. It is not an airy resolution for behind it lies a culture and understanding of the important role our legs play in our lives.

Many of us believe that our hands are the most important extension of our body. They are versatile and dextrous, able to per-form countless tasks. They make us different from most other living creatures. They give us distinction in the animal world. Our hands make us unique and special.

If we disregard our self-importance for a moment, we realize that this conclusion is incorrect. Our hands and arms may be very useful to us, but our legs are crucial. There are creatures in this world with only legs, whether in a pair or in great number, but there are no crea-tures with only hands.

Moving around is of primary importance. That is not an understatement. In the Chinese language, 'living creature' is written

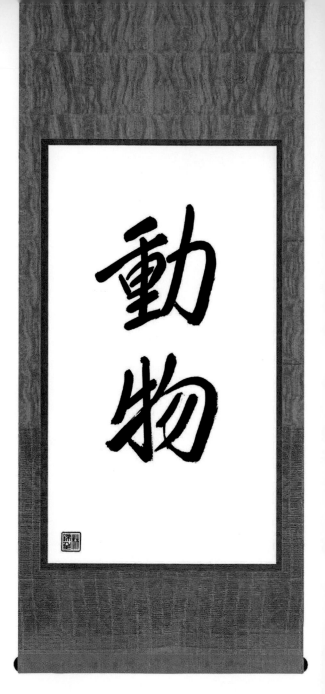

Above *The calligraphy for 'living creature' means 'thing that moves'.*

in two characters literally meaning, 'thing that moves'. Animals differ from inanimate objects because they can move at will.

In Chinese culture, basic human needs are listed as clothing, eating, sheltering, and travelling. Our legs are the bodily manifestation of travelling. However, our modern lifestyle has greatly reduced our opportunity to walk and our pleasure of walking. A few generations ago, walking was a major part of our lives, whether living in the city or the countryside.

The benefits of walking – and walking correctly – are reflected in Chinese folklore and many aspects of household wisdom.

Take a hundred steps after every meal and live to a hundred years.

However, this statement may be outdated. Since we are walking so little nowadays, we should be taking a thousand steps after each meal, not a hundred.

Our legs, and our ability to walk well, are a direct indicator of our mental and physical health. They are a dynamic part of our wellbeing. This is summarized by yet another example of ancient Chinese household wisdom:

Before the person grows old, the legs grow old.

Problems with the legs can be an early sign of ageing, and are undoubtedly a sign of a general decline in health. Deterioration, with complications, can start to happen at an early age, even to athletes and dancers.

Why is this so? What is the connection between legs and health? The answer is in the very nature of our limbs. Each morning as we get out of bed, our legs support our full weight and continue to do so, faithfully, throughout the day until we go to sleep. No other body part bears the same amount of prolonged physical stress continuously. It is no surprise that our legs are strongly linked to our wellbeing.

One branch of Chinese massage therapy, known in the West as reflexology, has gained much popularity in recent years. It is based on the principle that your health is reflected in the soles of your feet. Through pressure applied to acupoints on the feet, and various other techniques, therapeutic change can be brought about.

The walking systems of Chi Kung provide what our legs lack in modern life, building up greater strength and nourishing them with vitality and energy. These systems are methods of personal cultivation with their own discipline.

They are particularly beneficial to those people who under or overuse their legs. Those who are on their legs all day can use walking Chi Kung to 'tune' down their legs, while those who are sedentary most of their working day, can 'tune' up their legs. The direction of 'tuning' can go either way because the regular practice of Chi Kung is able to bring you back to natural balance, whatever your displacement may be.

Walking Chi Kung is also ideal for those students who are attracted to Chi Kung and Zhan Zhuang but, in their practice, find standing still a major challenge.

How to use this book

This is the first book in which I focus on Chi Kung in motion, and give the legs and walking the attention and recognition they deserve. It offers clear instructions for the walking systems of Chi Kung and its foundation training postures and techniques.

With detailed illustrations and a step-by-step text, readers should find this book both appealing and useful. The descriptions of the walking systems are not limited to just the physical choreography. I also describe the traditional mental and spiritual aspects of the movements so that, rather than performing the sequences in a mindless fashion, you will be able to practise them with some degree of understanding of the philosophy that underlies them.

All the instructions in this book are based not simply on the opinions of a single individual, but on the experiences and knowledge of many past masters across the ages. Follow them precisely and carefully and you will be in very safe hands. Do not try to mix different disciplines together or make variations of the exercises. Each instruction is carefully gauged and structured for your physical and mental wellbeing.

Part One introduces you to the art of natural and reverse breathing. Both are essential for your progress and development in the body arts.

Part Two helps you build a good physical foundation for the steps and walks that follow. It gives exercises for training and strengthening specific leg muscles, as well as standing postures. You should return to this section from time to time.

Part Three is the final phase of training before you start working on steps and walking systems. It is the stage where you progress from being stationary to moving. I explain the six directional forces that are the key to this leap.

FROM BONES TO PAPER

Chinese writing is thought to have been invented during the latter half of the second millennium BC, and to have evolved without evidence of foreign influence. The writing has undergone relatively little change since then. As a pictographic writing system, the characters were regarded as magical and sacred by the ancient Chinese, and were inscribed on animal bones and turtle shells for the purpose of divination and religious rituals. They are still used as a divinatory medium. The calligraphies shown here show the evolution of the Chinese character denoting 'leg'.

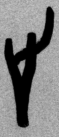

ORACLE BONE SCRIPT (Jia Gu Wen) Used during the Shang and Yin Dynasties, 1400–1200 BC. This character is one of several graphical variations of the foot image.

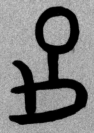

ORACLE BONE SCRIPT (Jia Gu Wen) This character, from the same period, seems to be derived from the foot image with an extension. Together, they represent the leg.

Part Four describes a variety of steps for you to study and learn. This is a special branch of the art of Da Cheng Chuan. The colourful steps are well illustrated and you are given careful instructions.

Part Five offers a number of complete walking systems that can be used independently. Their details and origins are colourful and inspiring. To practise them well takes time and dedication, so try to be patient.

In time, if you follow the book correctly, you should feel improvements in both your body and mind. Your legs will feel firmer and more vitalized, and your back will feel straighter and more supple. Your breathing will be deeper and stronger and you will also begin to feel warmer all over. You may notice an improvement in your mental abilities too, with an enhanced ability to focus on the task at hand. You will feel healthier and more relaxed. Most of all, you will feel fit – fitness

in the sense that your body is in a healthy and comfortable harmony with itself, rather than merely having the external appearance of physical fitness.

I hope that this book will open a door to a new understanding of the world and a new way of life, that, in turn, may lead to greater opportunities and prosperity.

Like knowing the destination before you embark on a long journey, you might like a glimpse of the forthcoming reward of this physical and mental expedition. The exercise shown over the next six pages, The Peacock Opens its Fan, is a telling sample of what you may accomplish with time, patience, and regular training.

At this stage, just read through the text. Aim to have this inspirational exercise as one of the last you will practise from this book. When you have achieved an adequate level of confidence with the steps, walks, and foundation training, return to this section and try this sequence.

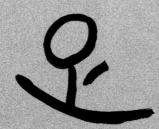

BRONZE SCRIPT (Jin Wen)
Used during the Zhou Dynasty, 1100–256 BC, this script was commonly used on bronze vessels. The writings were either directly cast with the vessels or inscribed later.

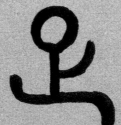

LESSER SEAL SCRIPT (Xiao Zhuan)
Different forms of Chinese writing were unified by the first emperor of China During the Qin Dynasty, 221–207 BC. Calligraphers still use the script in their name chops (seals).

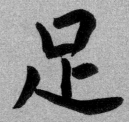

STANDARD SCRIPT (Kai Shu)
With the invention of paper and the use of brushes, Han Dynasty 207 BC –220 AD, characters became more linear to suit the new medium. This is the modern character for 'leg'.

The Peacock Opens its Fan

The mythical phoenix is a powerful and gracious creature, both admired and worshipped across many lands. In Chinese mythology, it is the female counterpart and companion of the dragon, Master of Water, and itself a Master of Fire. The peacock is the earthly reflection of the phoenix – a mortal avatar of its distant cousin in Heaven.

The elegant sequence of movements, shown here, draws inspiration from the splendid peacock with its expansive, glamorous tail and distinctively proud walk as he displays his magnificent attributes.

The graceful sequence characterizes the peacock's most distinctive feature: the opening of its incomparable tail feathers, shown by the upward rising and spreading of the arms. The peacock's strutting walk has been formalized into the outward kick of the foot, before it is carefully lowered to the ground.

The emulation is internal as well as external. When practising the exercise, you should try to exhibit a spiritual and mental portrayal of the peacock: its elegance, grace, and pride should radiate from your face. It is useful to think of the movement as a dance. Your motion should be smooth, slow, and rhythmic. Keep your knees relaxed throughout.

Do not be deceived by the elegance of the movement and consider the exercise weak and airy. Peacock tail feathers are a symbol of power and majesty. Your arms and hands, which mimick the tail feathers, should be equally powerful and splendid.

As you improve try, increasingly, to keep your head at the same level. This is more demanding than it appears but, as you put in more effort, so your movements will become more graceful and the labour more rewarding.

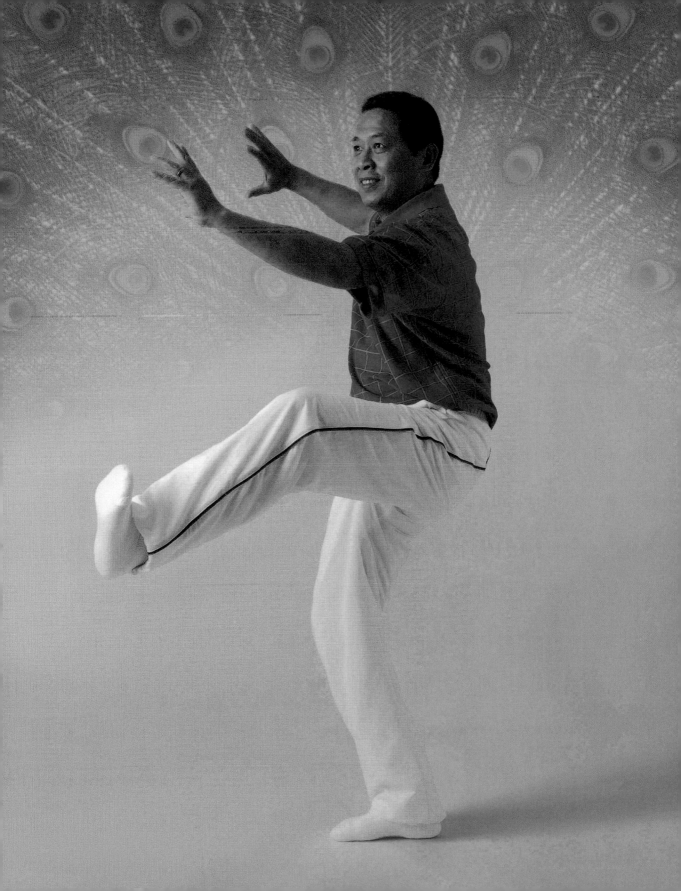

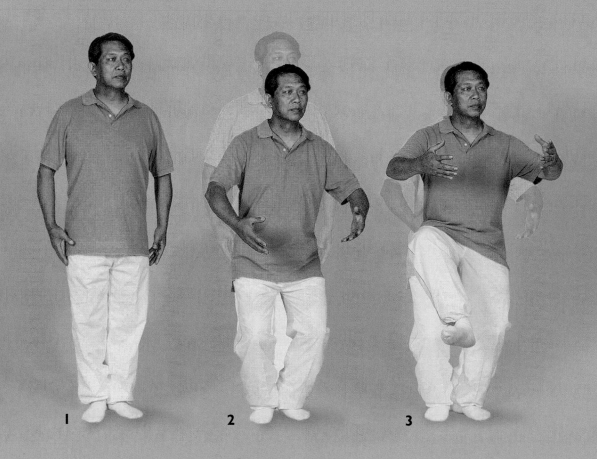

1 Begin with your heels together and toes apart at an angle of about 45 degrees. Stand straight but not rigid. Relax your hips, belly, and knees. Let your arms hang loosely from your shoulders with your palms facing your thighs. Have only a small space between your elbows and your sides and your fingers apart and slightly curved. Face forward and keep your neck and jaw loose. Breathe slowly and deeply through your nose.

2 Raise your hands slowly in front of you as if you are lifting a huge balloon. Bend both your knees and your hips slightly. Imagine you are sitting on an invisible stool or a huge balloon. Keep your eyes facing forward.

3 Shift your weight entirely to your left foot. Continue raising your hands to about the level of your shoulders and, as you do so, slowly lift your right knee with your foot flexed and still turned out. Avoid bending your elbows further and raising your knee too high.

4 Turn your torso and your gaze slightly to the right. Turn your palms outward and spread your hands out to the sides and up, drawing two smooth arcs in the air. Slightly straighten your raised leg out

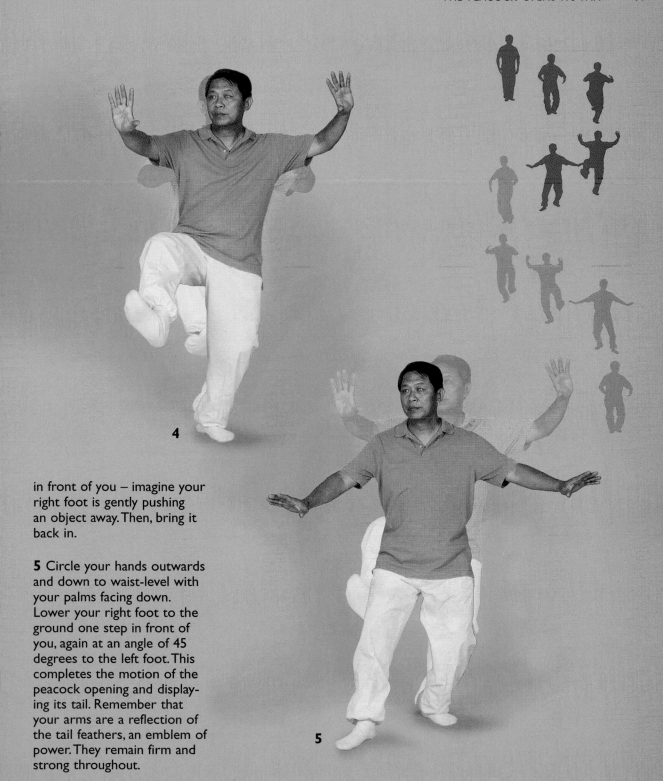

4

5

in front of you – imagine your right foot is gently pushing an object away. Then, bring it back in.

5 Circle your hands outwards and down to waist-level with your palms facing down. Lower your right foot to the ground one step in front of you, again at an angle of 45 degrees to the left foot. This completes the motion of the peacock opening and displaying its tail. Remember that your arms are a reflection of the tail feathers, an emblem of power. They remain firm and strong throughout.

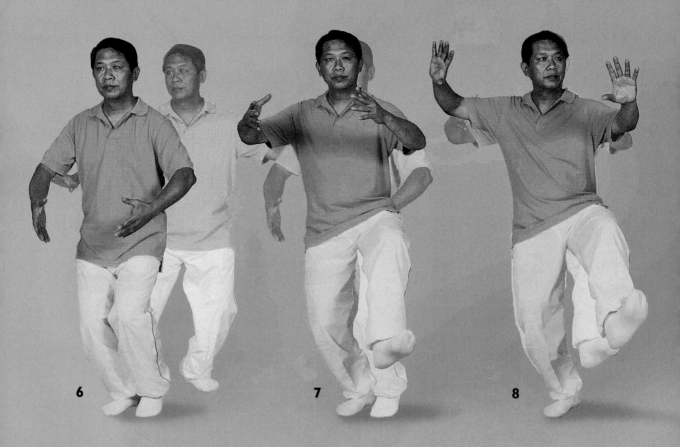

6

7

8

6 Slowly raise both your hands together in front of your belly, again as if lifting a hugh balloon. Draw your left foot forward and adjust your weight accordingly, sinking it into the right leg. Notice that your left leg is more bent than your right.

7 Lift your left knee and raise both arms, together, until the hands are approximately at the same level as your shoulders. Keep your arms in the same open position throughout this move.

8 Keeping your balance upright, turn your torso and gaze to the left. Your hands break from the balloon, as if it has just exploded, and fan out to either side. Press forward with your left foot, then withdraw. This is a mirror image of step 4.

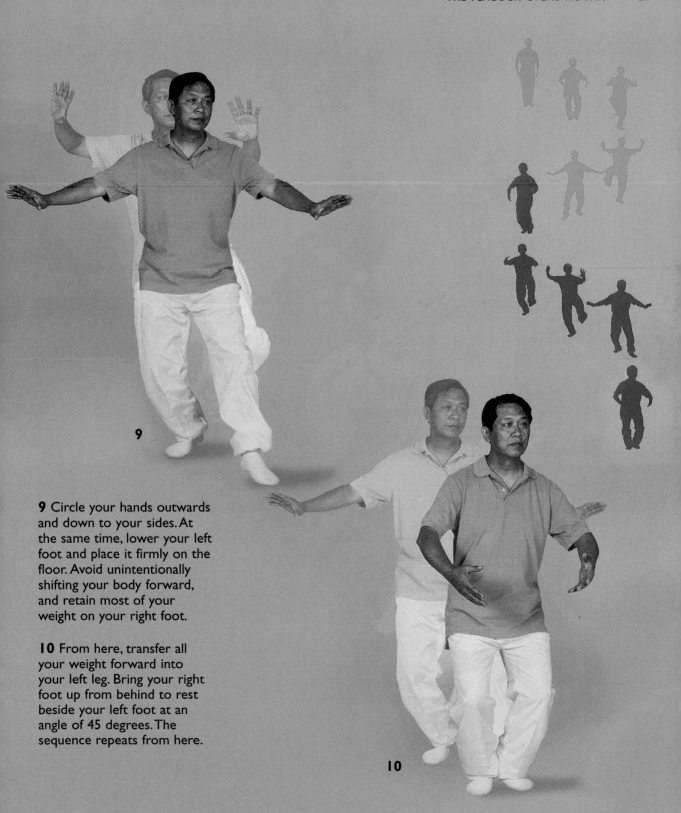

9 Circle your hands outwards and down to your sides. At the same time, lower your left foot and place it firmly on the floor. Avoid unintentionally shifting your body forward, and retain most of your weight on your right foot.

10 From here, transfer all your weight forward into your left leg. Bring your right foot up from behind to rest beside your left foot at an angle of 45 degrees. The sequence repeats from here.

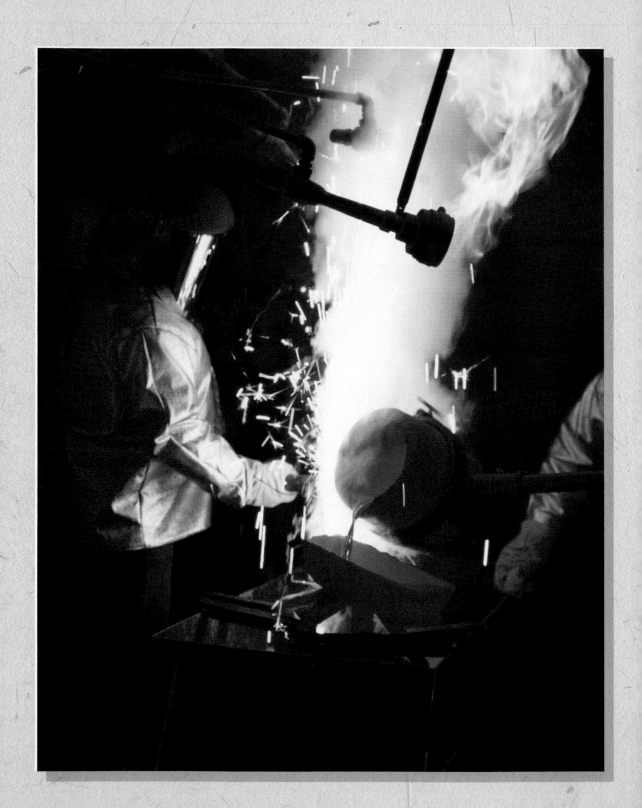

PART ONE

BREATHING ~ THE FURNACE WITHIN

You are going through a furnace:
everything mental and physical
is being tempered and moulded.

GRAND MASTER WANG XIANG ZHAI

The making of fire was probably mankind's first great creation. The furnace, in its various sizes, forms, and shapes is not just a heating system but a process of transformation and refinement of almost magical ability.

It serves many functions in society, appearing in various guises. In a smithy, the furnace is where raw materials are forged and tempered into powerful weapons and great works of art. In a herbalist's cauldron, the potent components of herbs are extracted. In a kitchen, the stove has for countless generations allowed cooks to transform basic ingredients into tasty cuisines. The combustion engine that runs most modern forms of transport is a mobile furnace propelling movement. These 'furnaces' may have different names, but they share the same underlying essence, and show the universality of the furnace throughout human civilization.

This insight did not escape the keen perception of past sages and wise men. They observed, understood, and embraced the idea, describing the world we live in as one great furnace, with the sky as the lid, the Earth as the base, and the myriad of things in the world as the contents.

Modern understanding of the world reinforces this model. The molten magma beneath the Earth's surface is the fire of the furnace, and the atmosphere is like the lid protecting us from cosmic radiation.

The concept of the furnace is not restricted to the external world. It can also be seen at an inner level. The human body is, itself, a complicated furnace, continuously transforming and refining you. In China, this process is known as internal alchemy.

In biology, the furnace idea is used to explain power generation within each cell, in specialized cell organelles, which are called mitochondria. These tiny structures are described as the 'boiler houses' of cells.

Breathing is one of the most critical and necessary functions of the human body. It is subtle, self-regulating, and unnoticeable most of the time, yet it is the key indicator of whether we are alive.

The art of breathing is extremely important, but often undervalued. Chi Kung is one of many Eastern systems that are globally recognized for their unique breathing methods. These breathing techniques have become a symbol of Eastern spiritualism.

However, some people have mistaken Chi Kung as nothing more than a set of breathing exercises. This is an incomplete and inaccurate interpretation of the art. It would be like saying that the ocean is merely a blue mass of water, while ignoring the billions of lives and mysteries it holds.

The contemporary Chinese character for Chi, the primal universal energy, is partly responsible for this misinterpretation. The ancient character, however, is a reminder of the ideology of Chi. The complete burning furnace is literally illustrated in brush-strokes to become a new word. It shows how reverently the Chinese hold this model, and how deeply they respect the furnace.

Mastering the art of breathing brings immense benefits. It is an art both vast and profound. Whether your goal is of a spiritual, martial, or medical nature, or just to achieve mental and psychological relaxation, you will find the art of breathing indispensable.

OXYGEN: FUELLING THE FIRE

The furnace is not just a colourful image passed on by our creative forefathers. It is a highly pragmatic model.

All mechanisms – technological, biological, or metaphorical – are made up of inputs, outputs, and processes. For you and me, human beings, and all air-breathing creatures, our first and foremost input is oxygen.

From the moment of birth, an infant's first act is to breathe. The first input is air. When a person dies, their last act is to take a final breath. A person's life is the continuity of breathing, the uninterrupted input of oxygen. We could say a person is a breathing machine.

It is possible for us to survive many days without food; a few days without water; but we cannot survive more than a few minutes without air.

You are fundamentally a flame that is fuelled by oxygen. Everything else is secondary. If the oxygen is cut off, the flame goes out. Once you acknowledge this, it is easy to understand your body, the human vessel, as a furnace. This is not an entirely new idea to Western minds; poets and writers, both past and present, often describe human life as a light or candle flame.

TAN TIEN – THE HUMAN CENTRE

Every object and every thing has a centre. Intuitively we know that every object can be characterized by a single point. That unique point is the centre. An object may be bent, chipped, or distorted, but as long as the centre remains intact, the object endures. It is only when the centre is destroyed that the object is truly gone.

The human body is no different. It has a centre that is the core of your physical and spiritual being. This centre is known as the Tan Tien (pronounced 'Dan Dyen'). It is sometimes known in the West as the 'Sea of Chi'. The Tan Tien is located about 3 cm (1¼ in) below your navel, approximately a third of the way into your body.

One interpretation of the Tan Tien is that it represents the physical 'centre of mass' of an average human being: an axis or pivot point of human flexibility. This is a highly practical interpretation in the world of martial arts.

Another perspective is that the Tan Tien is the nucleus and source of human life. In women, it is where new life is conceived and where new lives grow. In men, the Tan Tien is the inner extension, the virtual root, of the male reproductive organ. We can say, therefore, that the Tan Tien is the centre of human reproduction.

For internal alchemy, where the human body is one great, complex furnace, the Tan Tien is an elixir. The Chinese term, Tan Tien, literally means 'the field of elixir'. Here, it is the content that the human cauldron is cooking up. It is a field because it holds great potential and can be productively cultivated.

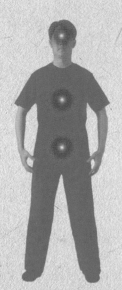

Higher Tan Tien

Middle Tan Tien

Lower Tan Tien

The human body can be viewed as having three sub-centres. They are known as the lower Tan Tien, the middle Tan Tien, and the higher Tan Tien. The lower Tan Tien is at the same point as the actual Tan Tien. The middle Tan Tien is located at the centre of your torso, behind the sternum. The higher Tan Tien lies deep within the head, behind the centre of your two eyebrows.

PREPARATION
Before beginning your breathing exercises, find a comfortable and private place in which to practise.

In ancient times, holy and wise men sought isolated places in the wilderness or high up in the mountains, for ideal conditions free of distraction. For us, however, in the modern world, a quiet room will suffice.

You may choose to put on some light background music for the duration of the breathing session or you may prefer to practise in complete silence. As many people find it difficult to relax when there is total silence, we recommend light background music. If external sounds are not too noisy or irritating, open your window slightly, allowing yourself access to fresh air. This makes a great difference.

When breathing with your lower or middle Tan Tien, you may do so standing up or sitting down. If you prefer standing, have your legs slightly bent and the feet apart at approximately the same width as your shoulders. If you prefer to sit, place an armless chair in or near the centre of the room away from any obstruction. Anything in the room that is annoying, irritating, or makes you feel disturbed, should be removed.

Sit squarely on the chair, in a relaxed and upright position. Do not cross your legs or have your knees together. Your legs should be parted at the same width as your shoulders, and your toes facing forward. Adjust the gap between your knees until your legs are at the most comfortable position.

If your chair has a back, do not rest against it. Have your upper body relaxed and upright, but not tense. Do not tilt forward or lean back, and keep your head facing forward at all times. Only when you feel relaxed, calm, and in harmony with yourself, should you start your breathing session.

Be aware that these are breathing exercises. Although they are complementary to meditations, it is important not to confuse the two. Resist the urge to mix any other disciplines into the following breathing practices at this stage. Your aim here is to build a strong foundation of good breathing. Without this, any future development in meditation will be hampered.

Natural breathing

Breathing exercises are a workout that can refine the human centre – the Tan Tien. They are a process of cultivating the whole being, bringing it to equilibrium.

Note that the word equilibrium is used instead of balance, as you are not seeking static balance but a dynamic stability, even when everything is in fluid motion.

Natural breathing is not something that we need to learn because it is already built in to the human system since birth. Why then are there so many great schools of breathing and meditation techniques? The answer is that we forget how to breathe naturally as we grow up, and need to rediscover our rhythm of natural breathing.

As infants we breathe naturally; each breath is deep, gentle, slow, and even. Our breathing rhythm is suited to our needs, and optimal for general health.

As we grow to adulthood many things distract and divert our lives from a healthy path. Our breathing may become fast, short, or shallow, immensely different from how we used to breathe when we were infants.

Our natural breathing rhythm has given way to our stressful lifestyles. Whether from staying out late having fun, or from long periods of hard work, our body and mind are very often full of tension. We may find that even in our sleep, it is difficult for us to truly rest. Our present form of breathing is the result of such restlessness.

To return to health, we need to breathe naturally again. Fortunately, natural breathing is not lost to us, only hidden – buried away by years of neglect. With dedicated practice and patience, our natural breathing can be rediscovered. In turn, this will bring us a healthy mind, body, and spirit.

THE HIGHER TAN TIEN

This particular sub-centre, the higher Tan Tien, is not part of the breathing system of this or the following section. There are some important differences between this sub-centre and the other two. The lower and middle Tan Tiens are associated with your energy and Chi. They are the sub-centres of power and life force, relating to your physical being.

On the other hand, the higher Tan Tien is associated more with your mental and spiritual self. It is the nucleus of your conscious and sub-conscious mind. It is located between the two eyebrows, halfway into the head.

The higher Tan Tien can be understood in many different ways. One of its most famous expressions is as the mind's eye. In the East, there are many sources of literature describing the cultivation and inner working of the mind's eye. Many gods of Eastern religions are depicted showing a physical manifestation of a third eye as a sign of mastery of their higher Tan Tien. However, such literature falls beyond the scope of this book.

Natural chest breathing ~ middle Tan Tien

Raise your hands in front of you level with your chest. Let the arms form a circle as if you are gently embracing some-one. Avoid having your elbows stick out too far or having them too bent. A natural, comfortable angle is best.

Breathe slowly and gently through your nose, keeping your mouth shut. Let your eyelids lower, but keep the eyes open. Allow your body to dictate the rhythm of your breathing as that will be the natural rhythm. It should be gentle but deep, slow but long.

Let your chest expand as you inhale, and relax as you exhale. As you inhale, let each breath travel down to the natural breathing centre of your chest. You may be able to recognize it, intuitively, as you breathe. It is located within the chest approximately level with where your ribs join the sternum. This point is known as the middle Tan Tien.

Begin your practice with sessions of two minutes. As you improve, build up gradually to five minutes.

1 Imagine that the middle Tan Tien is an energy point. As you inhale, the breath travels down to your middle Tan Tien and your chest expands. The point of energy enlarges into a sphere encompassing your entire chest.

2 As you exhale, relax your chest. The energy sphere returns to a single point.

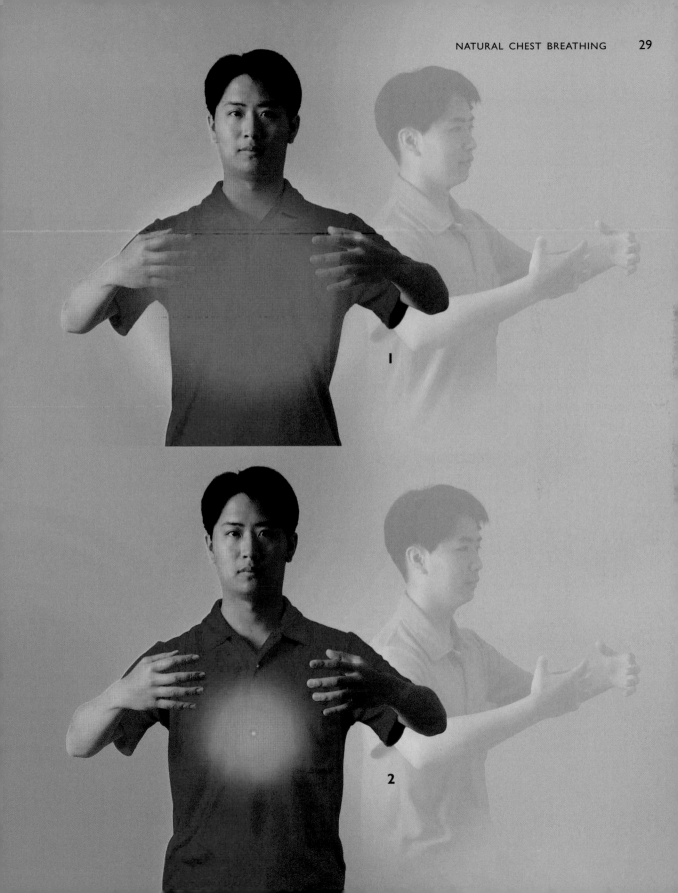

1

2

Natural belly breathing ~ lower Tan Tien

This breathing exercise focuses on the lower Tan Tien. Presented here as a standing practice, it can also be a sitting practice, if you prefer. The lower Tan Tien is located identically to the Tan Tien of the full body (see page 26).

Place your hands in front of your lower abdomen as if you have lowered your arms to rest a little after the previous breathing exercise – Natural Chest Breathing ~ middle Tan Tien. Imagine that you have a large belly under which your hands are resting. The palms face diagonally in-ward, fingers apart and slightly curved. Do not have your arms too close to your body; give yourself space between your elbows and your sides; relax your shoulders; and do not let your body tilt forward or back.

With your mind calm and body relaxed, breathe in gently and deeply through your nose. Let your breath travel all the way down from your nose to your lower Tan Tien in one smooth, clear passage. It is a long way down, so you must coordinate the depth and length of your breath accordingly. Let there be a point of energy at your lower Tan Tien.

Begin your practice with sessions of two minutes. As you improve, build up gradually to five minutes.

1 As you inhale, the breath expands your belly. As it does so, the energy point expands into a sphere filling your belly.

2 When you exhale, the energy sphere shrinks back to a point. You could imagine that the energy sphere is a balloon inflating and deflating.

The depth and length of your exhalations should be the same as your inhalations. Let your body guide the rhythm of your breath.

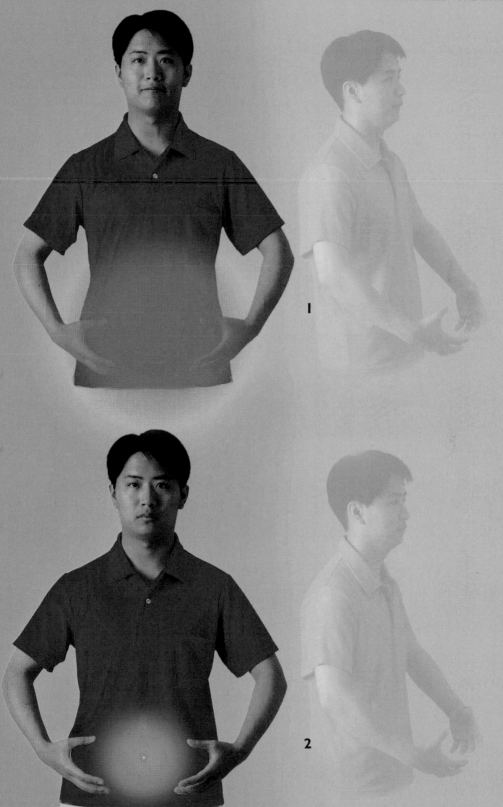

1

2

Full body natural breathing ~ full body Tan Tien

In the previous two breathing exercises, the focus has been on a particular part of the body. You could practise them either sitting down or standing up. To breathe with your whole body, however, you must stand up.

Here, you align your three sub-centres (your higher, middle, and lower Tan Tiens) into one singular centre, the Tan Tien (see pages 25–26). It encompasses and reflects your entire body. Compared with breathing into the lower Tan Tien, the difference is one of scale and magnitude.

The famous posture shown here, is known as the position of supreme emptiness. Its Chinese name is Wu Chi and it is also known as the position of primal energy. A fuller and more detailed elaboration is laid out on pages 56–57.

Just as before, inhale through your nose. Notice that your breath needs to go a long way down to your Tan Tien. This is why you need to breathe slowly and deeply.

You can practise this exercise for as long as you feel comfortable, but do not push yourself too hard. It is, after all, meant to be a relaxing practice.

WU CHI
Here is a brief guideline to standing in Wu Chi correctly.

Stand upright with your legs at approximately shoulder-width apart and your feet facing forward.

Let your arms dangle loosely at your sides.

Relax the knees and elbows so that they are not locked into a straight position.

Avoid tilting forward or leaning backward.

Relax all your muscles.

1 Imagine that your centre is a point of energy at the Tan Tien. Every time you breathe in, let the point inflate like a balloon. The point expands into a perfect sphere, which encompasses your entire body and beyond. Your arms move away from the body slightly as if expanding with the sphere. However, this movement is negligible, more mental than physical.

2 As you breathe out your sphere reduces to a single point and your arms gently return to their original positions.

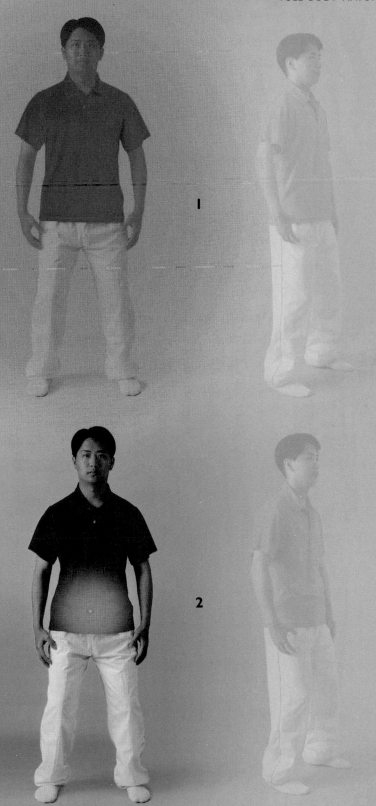

1

2

Reverse breathing

At first glance, reverse breathing may appear to conflict with the concept given in the previous section, but this is not so. As you are seeking a state of equilibrium, you must breathe in a natural rhythm that your body recognizes. However, a state of equilibrium is not limited to a single breathing rhythm. The other breathing rhythm that can achieve this state is called reverse breathing.

A simple analogy explains how this, apparently conflicting idea, can be true. Imagine trying to place a smooth ball on a hill. Whichever part of the hillside you place the ball, it will start rolling. The ball is not at rest; it is in disequilibrium and will move until it finds balance. We know that, at the bottom of the hill, the ball will rest. This is its natural position of equilibrium where gravity has helped it to settle. However, there is another position where the ball can be at rest – at the very peak of the hill!

The system of reverse breathing is like a ball on the peak of the hill. It is counter-intuitive to your breathing rhythm and, therefore, without your natural instinct to guide you, it is harder to master. The ball on top of the hill, has worked against gravity to acheive its climb. Similarly, reverse breathing is more demanding and, therefore, more advanced than natural breathing.

Another major difference between natural breathing and reverse breathing is the involvement of your willpower. Here, in the reverse breathing exercises, the rhythm of your breath disagrees with the rhythm of your body. You need to engage your will-power to make the two rhythms cooperate with each other. However, try to keep your mind relaxed and at ease at all times.

In practice, you have probably experienced more reverse breathing, in the course of your daily lives, than you realize. Every time you open a bottle, or fix a screw into a hard object, you are doing a crude form of reverse breathing.

The preparation for this breathing session is the same as before. Find a quiet room free from distractions. Open the window so you can have access to fresh air.

If you plan to sit, choose a chair with no arms and place it in the centre of the room. Sit with your back erect but relaxed. Your knees are parted at about the same width as your shoulders. Your feet point forward. Do not let your body sway to the front or the back, the left or the right.

Face forward but keep your neck loose and relaxed. Let all the tensions in your mind and muscles wash away as if you were being cleansed by a river flowing over you.

When you have done all of the above, it is time to start your breathing practice.

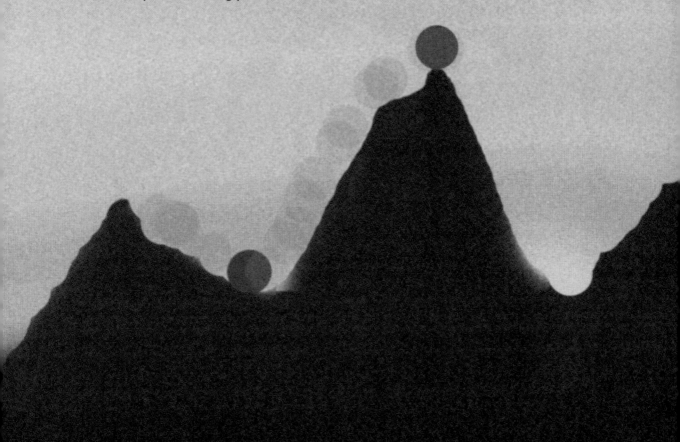

Reverse chest breathing ~ middle Tan Tien

Position your hands in front of your body at the same level as your chest and approximately shoulder-width apart. Your palms face down and your fingers forward. Your arms should only be moderately curved and your elbows should not stick out too much.

Breathe in and out through your nose. Let your breath be long, slow, and subtle. Remember that you are breathing with your chest and that the centre point is the middle Tan Tien. Once again, while you are breathing, imagine that there is an energy sphere expanding and shrinking.

Start with two-minute breathing sessions. As you improve, build up slowly and gradually.

1 As you inhale, guide the air down to your middle Tan Tien while compressing your chest. Imagine that your energy sphere is collapsing or crystallizing into a highly charged and powerful energy point.

2 When you exhale, relax your chest and let that powerful energy point disperse into a perfect sphere with a diameter equalling your chest.

Please note *When you inhale, do not compress your chest so much that it hurts. Avoid putting too much effort into the visualization otherwise your mind and body will become tense.*

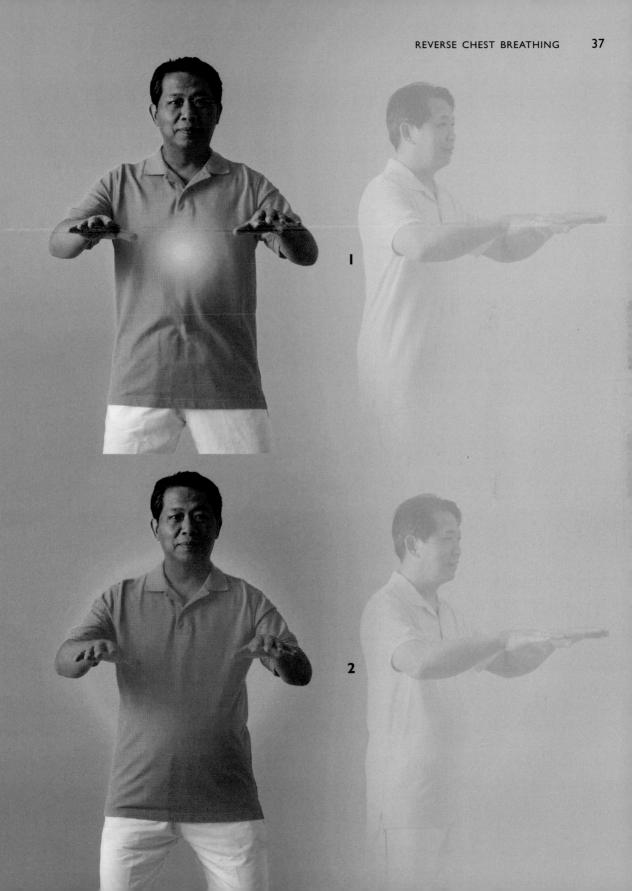

1

2

Reverse belly breathing ~ lower Tan Tien

After completing the previous exercise, Reverse Chest
Breathing ~ middle Tan Tien, lower your arms so that your
hands are level with your waist. Again, your elbows should
not stick out too far – your arms should curve naturally.
Avoid having them too close to your body otherwise your
shoulders will stiffen. Turn your hands in slightly, and then
start reverse breathing again.

Breathe with your lower Tan Tien through your nose.
Keep your lips firmly sealed, but do not tense your jaw. Your
breath should travel smoothly and freely in and out of the
lower Tan Tien. Remember, also, that in this exercise you have
a choice of standing up or sitting down.

Start with two-minute breathing sessions. Then, as you
improve, slowly and gradually build up these sessions.

1 Squeeze your belly in as
you inhale. Remember that
the centre of your breathing
is in the lower abdomen, the
lower Tan Tien. Do not place
too much emphasis on the
top half of your belly. Let
your imaginary energy ball
condense as if it were a
planet collapsing against its
own mass. Avoid squeezing
your belly too much.

2 Exhale slowly and let your
belly relax gradually, not in
one swift move as if dropping
a sack to the ground. Your
belly should not 'pop' out as
you exhale. Let your energy
point expand gradually at a
constant rate.

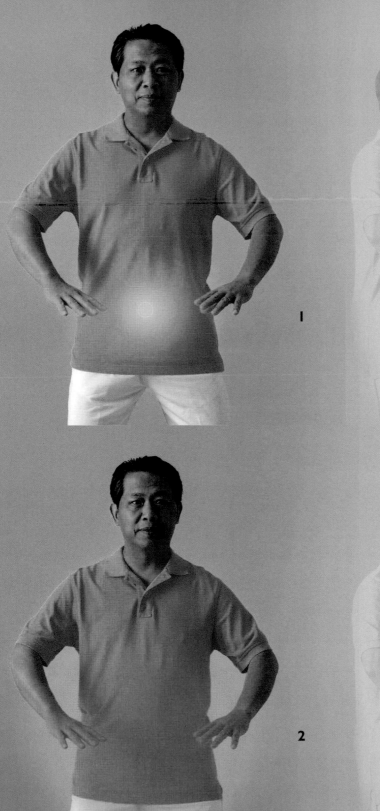

1

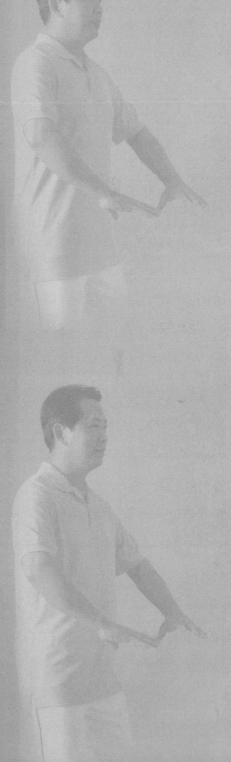

2

Full body reverse breathing ~ full body Tan Tien

This breathing exercise involves the most movement of all the breathing exercises in this section of the book. To breathe with your full body, you must stand up rather than sit.

Please remember the following key points when you stand for this exercise: keep your head facing forward; your legs shoulder-width apart, knees unlocked; palms facing down; and fingers straight. Try to relax all your muscles.

Imagine that your energy is all around you, both within you and beyond the surface of your body. It envelops you like a warm and subtle gaseous cocoon.

Begin with a session of two minutes and progress from there as you improve.

1 As you breathe in, collect the surrounding energy toward your Tan Tien. The energy travels down from above through your head, and up from the ground through your legs. Your lower belly contracts slightly as you inhale. Your hands rise up to chest-level as if they had floated up, light as feathers.

2 As you breathe out and you relax your belly, the energy disperses out in the same way it came in, returning to the ground below and air above. Lower your hands as if you are very gently pressing something down.

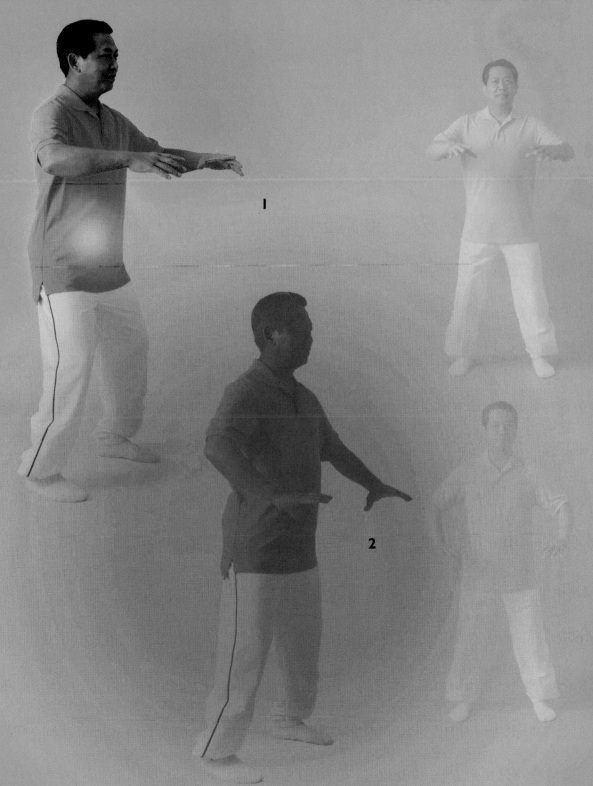

FREQUENCY OF PRACTICE

Natural breathing and reverse breathing systems are counterparts of each other, like Yin and Yang, mutually existing in opposite ways. In the beginning, practise only the three forms of natural breathing. Once you become familiar with, and confident of, your natural breathing skills, then you can start to practise the reverse breathing exercises.

Unlike other physical exercises, natural breathing techniques do not have an upper practice limit. There can be no such thing as breathing too much. You only go wrong if you breathe incorrectly. The main limitation here actually comes from your body — namely, the difficulty of the postures.

Reverse breathing, however, does have restrictions. There is a limit to how long your counter-intuitive rhythm can hold. Your willpower and concentration will ebb. When that happens, your breathing rhythm falters and you must stop. It takes time to rediscover natural breathing, and even longer to learn reverse breathing. Your body, especially your arms, become tired if you practise too long. It is best to practise your breathing exercises for two minutes daily, and gradually build up the duration of your sessions.

You can do these exercises whenever the need arises. They are excellent for calming nerves, relieving stress, refreshing the mind, and relaxing muscles. You can practise anytime of day whenever you feel stressed, nervous, or tired. They also make excellent preparation for studying or working.

You can adjust your breathing practice according to your lifestyle, and integrate it into your daily routine. As long as you practise correctly and regularly, you will become aware of an impressive difference. Correct breathing brings a greater supply of oxygen into your system.

BREATHING AND MEDITATION

It is not possible to mention breathing exercises without some small reference to meditation. The two are so intertwined that they are often mistaken for each other. On the outside, they appear virtually identical, their interrelationships are strong, but the gap between them is immense.

Meditation is a vast and wide-ranging subject encompassing many different schools of thought. In the West, the varied meditation disciplines are often confusingly lumped together under the one title, meditation. In the East, however, meditation is described by a variety of different names, offering us an insight into the various functions and underlying philosophies of each.

One title conveys forgetfulness: its objective being the unification of the self and Heaven. Another, described by Zen buddhists, suggests an interaction and understanding of the mysteries, the wordless wisdom of their doctrines. It is a cultivation of the heart and soul. In medicine, the name given to their meditation speaks of tranquillity and calm. In yet another field, meditation addresses the elusive Chi.

When you see them in this light, you realize that meditation and the breathing arts are not two distinct units, but separate parts of the same journey.

Breathing complements meditation, that is clear. Correct breathing is the stepping-stone to effective meditation; one is the foundation of the other. However, the link between the two is an elusive art. You should not randomly mix and match breathing exercises with meditations.

The topic of meditation is like a king whose kingdom has numerous states and provinces. As such, It is not possible to fit this vast and colourful sphere of knowledge within the breadth of these pages.

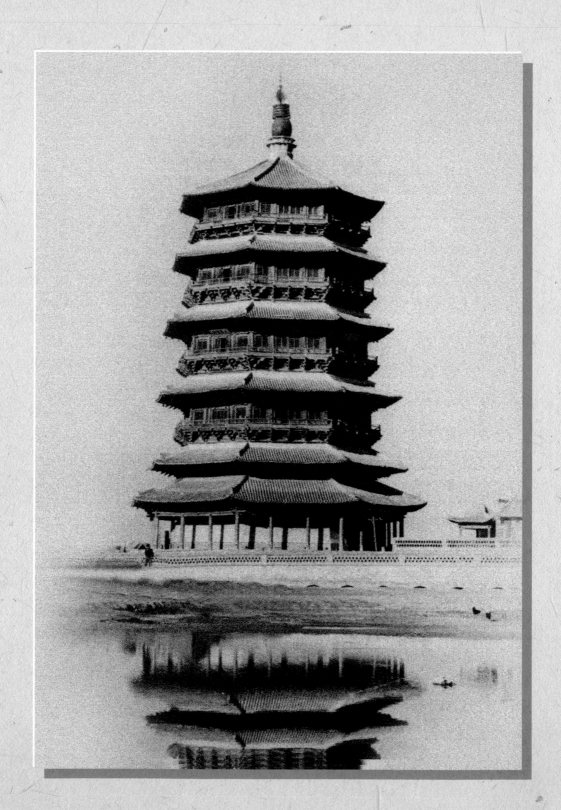

PART TWO

BUILDING THE FOUNDATION

The philosophy of building or creating anything can be summed up in one word: foundation. It is a simple word yet, with it, comes the wisdom of age and experience.

Creating or developing anything is like building a house. Most things are built from the ground upward; rarely the other way around. The foundation of any structure is of unequivocal importance. The base is always at least as large as the top, if not larger. Rarely, will you find a structure where the top is greater than the base.

Pyramids are excellent examples of this idea. The cross section of a pyramid gets progressively bigger toward the base. It is no wonder they have outlasted other ancient buildings, and rank among the great wonders of the world. Pyramids are based on a universal principle and are, therefore, found in both the Old and the New Worlds.

Lowering the centre of mass is the key to steadiness, firmness, and stability. It is the enigma behind the pyramids. Despite their greatness, pyramids are only an architectural metaphor for something deeper.

The same principle manifests with regard to humility and modesty. Lowering the ego and sense of self-importance makes you more steadfast and resolute. Only by being humble can a person truly make progress. This is one of the reasons why humility is so revered in spiritual practice.

All forms of human cultivations – whether of the mind or body – are based on this ideology. Education, the cultivation of knowledge, is an excellent example. In the early stages of education you study a wide variety of subjects. Only after proving that you have gained an adequate understanding of the subjects, by taking exams, do you proceed to higher education. As you progress upward through the educational system, the range of subjects studied becomes narrower. You become more specialized.

This principle also applies to your body. As you strengthen your lower limbs – your legs – you strengthen your whole self. In China, there is an apt role model called Bei Tao Yung, 'The old man who never falls'. This traditional toy is a hollow, wooden doll with a round base and a smaller top, on which is painted an image of an old man. A weight placed in the base means that no matter how you tilt or push the toy, it rebounds. This toy is a household symbol of tenacity, resolution, and dedication. Many parents teach their children to follow Bei Tao Yung's stable and rebounding qualities.

This section of the book focuses on building the foundations of good practice. These basic exercises may seem simple but, with dedication and consistent practice, they enable great progress during the later stages of your training.

Chinese traditional toys: an old man and woman who never fall down.

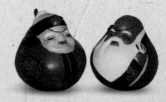

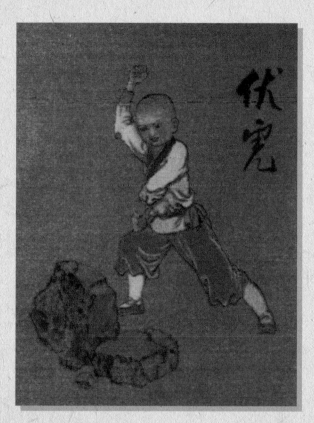

Left *This illustration, from the main frieze at the Shaolin temple in the Sung Mountains of Central China, shows a student practising the stance called 'Taming the Tiger'.*

STANCES

The first exercise for your foundation training is known as a stance. Stances are stationary postures frequently practised by martial artists. They are taught in various schools and disciplines of the martial arts. In fact the system of stances is one of the few common denominators shared between martial art disciplines. Stances are used as foundation training in all of them.

Stances are a set of postures or exercises that concentrate mainly on the legs. One example, called 'horse stance', is named after the posture one takes when riding a horse – it is adopted in the exercise shown on pages 48–49.

Although both systems are stationary, you must not confuse stances with Zhan Zhuang (see page 10). There is a vast internal difference between the two that sets them apart like an abyss. Both systems share stillness, but stance work focuses on framework and structure. The depth and format of the two systems cannot be compared.

Stance work trains the human body from an architectural and physical point of view. You could even say that stance work is technical in character.

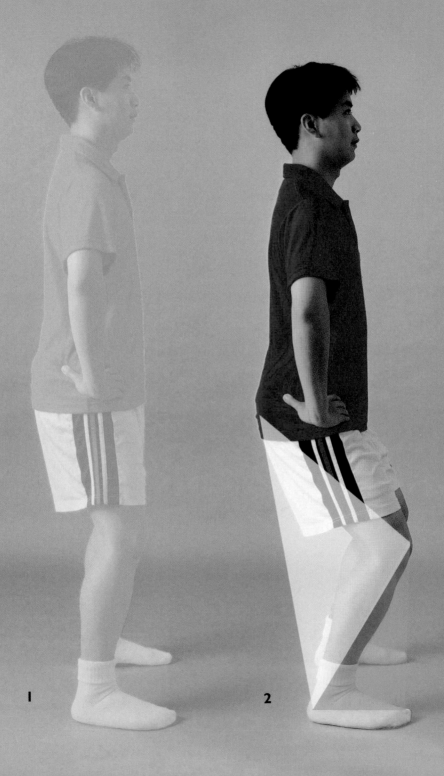

1

2

Strengthening the legs

Here is a stance to train your thigh muscles. Unlike most of the other exercises in this book, there is neither visualization nor any form of mental involvement. It is a subtle physical training upon the framework of the legs.

This exercise is mechanical artwork, aligning the toes, heels, knees, and hips. It is a structure of lines, triangles, and axes. Between the toes, heels, and knees, there is a rigid and architecturally powerful right-angled triangle. Between your heels, knees, and hips, there is another triangle. These subtle inner triangles are the underlying basis to building strength.

1 Stand upright with your legs slightly bent, and your head facing forward. Rest your hands on your hips, and avoid stiffening your shoulders. Do not stick out your bottom or tilt your body forward. Try to relax all your muscles and breathe calmly.

2 Slowly lower yourself by sinking your weight. Imagine you are sitting on an invisible stool. Bend your knees slightly but do not let them stick out further than your toes. Everything above your hips should remain unchanged. Keep your legs relaxed and stay in this position for about three minutes.

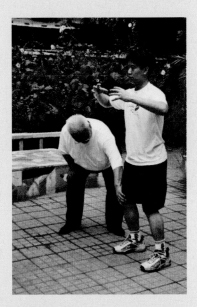

Above *Professor Yu checks the optimal position of Tinhun Lam's knees for a standing posture. He is making sure that the knees do not protrude over the toes.*

Training the muscles

In this exercise we focus on the calf muscles rather than the thighs. This stance requires more balancing skill, but the raised arms help support you, as well as being an aspect of the training.

Hold this position for as long as you can, and try to relax your entire body throughout the exercise. The calf muscles do not require your conscious attention during this exercise. You should not overexert yourself at any time. If you feel tired or start to lose your balance, lower your heels and stand up. Return to the initial position, rest for a moment, and then continue.

1 Raise your arms up to the sides and flex your wrists to tilt your hands up. Do not flex them so far that they hurt. Keep your fingers closed and straight. Imagine you are in a small alleyway pushing against both walls. Your shoulders should not be raised or stiff. Stand with your legs approximately shoulder-width apart, as illustrated by the pair of yellow lines.

2 Slowly lower your height and bend your knees while lifting both heels off the floor very slightly. Seek a delicately balanced position where you can be perfectly still. Your legs should be slightly squeezed inward as if you are holding a large balloon between your knees. Avoid leaning forward.

As you can see, there is a clear structure within this stance. The shoulders and wrists form a solid horizontal line supported by strong vertical lines through the toes, knees, and shoulders.

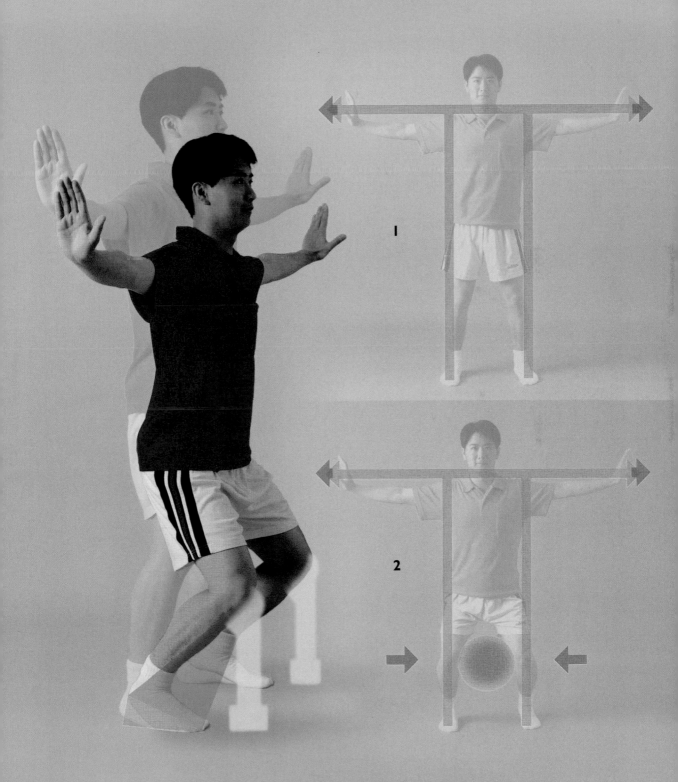

1

2

Second voluntary movements

With this leg exercise we focus, once again, on the calf muscles. This is by no means accidental. As we are focusing on our lower body, the legs, so, in turn, we pay greater attention to the lower parts of them.

The human body is truly an amazing structure. Its variety of muscles has given us such dexterity and flexibility that we have taken it very much for granted. Nevertheless, the differences between the muscles and their movements are vast. However, rather than dwelling on the many categories and mechanisms of muscles known in modern anatomy, our focus here is on the voluntary movements of certain muscles in our legs.

By voluntary movement, we refer to the contraction and relaxation of muscles that we can consciously control, as opposed to an involuntary muscle, such as our heart, which pumps faithfully and continuously whether we want it to or not.

Some voluntary movements of the muscles offer physical displacement. Moving the arms and legs are excellent examples of this. In this art, these muscle contractions are called the 'first voluntary movements'. By contracting and loosening various muscles, certain parts of the body will shift spatially.

These muscle contractions correspond to our daily body movements.

In this exercise, our attention falls more specifically on the 'second voluntary movements'. This term refers to movements of muscles that can contract and relax at our will, but offer no physical displacement – in other words, our body parts do not move. People are unaware of these movements because, in our everyday lives, we only consciously contract muscles for external or spatial reasons.

The second voluntary movements may appear inconsequential and meaningless at first but, with time and experience, you will realize that they are actually of monumental importance. Such muscle contractions are much more difficult to achieve than you might first realize. The mental effort and will-power needed are immense and exhausting.

In this exercise, you will be training one leg at a time. Unlike the previous two work-outs, the mental strength involved in this exercise is substantial. In the beginning, you will certainly find concentrating on these muscle movements strenuous and tiring. The aim here is to develop the second voluntary movements of your legs.

Please note *you are trying to bring the back-stage contractions of the calf muscles into conscious action. You can see, in the close-up illustrations of the leg (see facing page), that this exercise is subtle but very powerful. You should not engage any muscles above the knee or below the ankle. The reasoning behind this training is deeply and powerfully structured.*

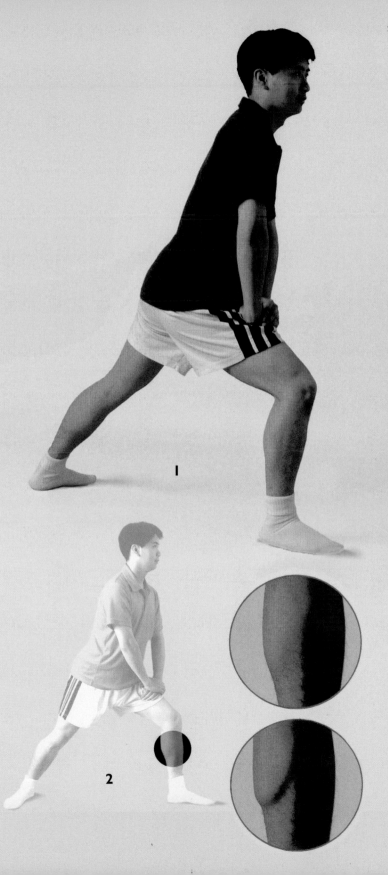

1 Take a large step forward with the right foot. The right leg is bent with the toes facing forward. The left leg remains straight, but the foot points slightly to the left. Avoid taking a step so large that it overstretches and hurts your inner thighs. That is not the objective.

Allocate 70 per cent of your weight on the right leg, and 30 per cent on the left. Rest both hands on your right thigh, near the hip, with the left hand on top. Contract your right calf muscles for as long as you can. When you reach the limit, relax the leg and start again. Repeat 30 times.

2 Switch to the other set of calf muscles. Your left leg is now bent and your right leg is straight. The left hand is sandwiched between the right hand and the left thigh. Tighten your left calf muscles for as long as possible before loosening again. Repeat 30 times.

Left *These two images show the calf muscles relaxed (top) and contracted (below).*

THE TRAINING

The particular training and ideology of the second voluntary movements were developed by Professor Yu Yong Nian, a disciple of the prominent Grand Master Wang Xiang Zhai, after many years of dedicated research.

The set of calf muscles is one of the least recognized parts of the human body. The calves are structurally important, of course, but they are more in the background than in the spotlight of our mind. They react to external circumstances rather than enacting upon them, and the many different layers of calf muscles are not all efficiently used. Our goal in this aspect of our training is to draw their full potential to the surface, as far as possible. That is the objective of training the second voluntary movements.

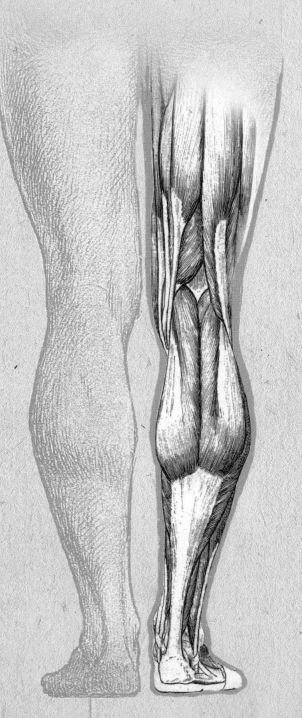

THE SECOND HEART

Our wellbeing is directly linked to good blood circulation. The core of our circulation is the heart, responsible for pumping blood throughout the numerous arteries, veins, and intricate capillary networks in the body.

As you would expect, the further away from the core something is, the weaker it gets. Our limbs are extensions of our body, and at the furthest reaches of our limbs are our feet. Hence, blood circulation is weakest there. The blood in your lower limbs needs to travel over 1 m (3¼ ft) to get back to the heart. In addition, when you are standing, the flow has to work against gravity. It is no surprise that circulation is weak in the feet — you know this to be true by experience. Whenever you are cold, your toes and fingers are the first to feel it. They have less access to your blood and energy circulations. The toes especially, are the first to get frostbite in winter.

Training the calf muscles takes time and dedication. It may be a little dry and bland on occasions, but the reasons and explanations behind this training are intriguing. The human heart is a coordinated system of muscles pumping blood around the body. Our hearts are essentially muscles. The fascinating thing about this concept is that you can also perceive this notion in the other direction: our muscles can serve as hearts.

Blood is pumped from the heart to the body extremities. On its return to the heart, blood travels under less pressure, as well as passing through veins that have no muscular tension of their own. Upward flow of the blood can be encouraged by the squeezing action of the muscles next to veins.

Your two sets of calf muscles can serve as efficient pumps for your blood circulation. Through training, your legs can voluntarily enhance circulation as if they were two great motor pumps, literally squeezing the blood up through the veins in your legs and feet. They ease the burden that your heart bears, offering you considerable relief. This is especially helpful to those who are troubled by heart problems. Personally, I have termed these calf muscle trainings, 'the second heart exercises'.

A chain is only as strong as its weakest link.

This simple epigram explains perfectly how the second heart can directly influence your health and inner power. Here, strength is not built upon other strengths; it is built on our weakness. By strengthening our weaker parts, we become fundamentally stronger. The baseline of our inner strength is raised. The weakest point of our circulation becomes a key to achieving greater energy and vitality. Our weakness becomes our strength.

Wu Chi

Body as the string lifts
Two eyes, the spiritual light, reserve;
Two ears listen to Supreme Tranquillity
The small belly is constantly round.

GRANDMASTER WANG XIANG ZHAI

This is a powerful position with which you must become familiar. Whether you are very experienced or just beginning Chi Kung, this posture should never be treated lightly or, worse, dismissed casually. You have already experienced Wu Chi, earlier, when practising full body natural breathing.

Wu Chi is the fundamental posture, the primal position. It is the alpha and the omega. The Chinese term means 'supreme emptiness'. As all things come from nothing and return to nothing, this posture therefore manifests the elusive beginning and end – like a circle.

This position emulates emptiness and, in doing so, it simultaneously encompasses everything in the universe. The Wu Chi posture is an alignment of energies between Heaven, Earth, and yourself. This is why it is also known as the position of primal energy. As Heaven refers to all things above, and Earth to all things below, this position links you, universally, to every other existing thing, as if part of a great chain. It allows you to recognize yourself as an integral part of myriad existence.

For those acquainted with Tai Chi Chuan, Wu Chi is a familiar sight. It is the posture at the beginning and end of the form. The implications of this are tremendous. Tai Chi Chuan is composed of colourful and inspiring movements, all belonging to the realm of existence illustrating that from nothingness myriad things come forth and eventually return to nothingness. Existence is but a momentary presence within the continuity of the void.

Wu Chi is a multi-layered concept, deep with wisdom. When practising, there is no need to dwell on its profound meaning otherwise your mind will become clouded. It is, however, helpful to recognize the depth of Wu Chi.

Standing in Wu Chi
Imagine you are standing outside in the rain. Each raindrop washes down over the contours of your body to the ground, washing away tension and anxiety, cleansing your mind and spirit.

Gaze forward and slightly down as if you are on the top of a mountain staring at the horizon. You are looking at nothing yet seeing everything. Relax your eyelids, but do not shut them. If you find this challenging, look out of your window and focus on something green and, preferably, natural, such as a tree.

Have your legs apart at approximately the same width as your shoulders, feet parallel, pointing forward.

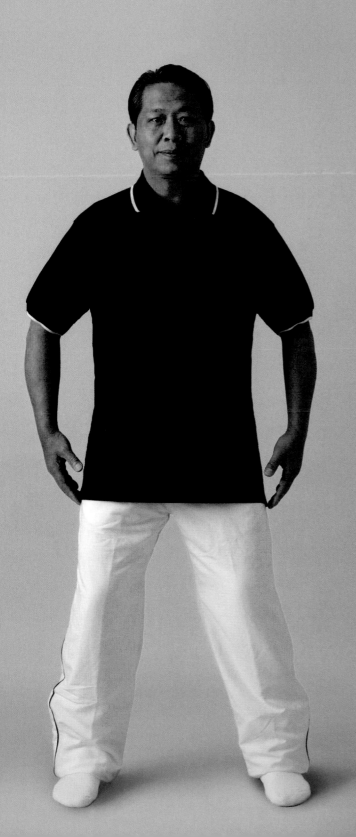

Let your arms hang gracefully from your shoulders, with a natural outward curve and a little space under the armpits.

Unlock your knees and elbows so that your limbs are not stiff and straight.

Maintain your body upright. Do not let it tilt forward or backward.

Sink your weight a little, as if you are sitting on a huge balloon.

Imagine you are being lifted by a golden thread from the top of your head. Relax all your muscles.

Practise this position for about five minutes each day. As you progress, build up gradually to ten minutes.

Understanding your centre

Standing is the most natural position recognized by the body. When standing, all your inner channels and circulations are aligned in the smoothest and most agreeable way. Nothing is folded, bent, or twisted. The flow of Chi and other body circulations are optimized.

The first and foremost standing position is Wu Chi (see pages 56–57). It is fundamentally integrated into your system. When you acheive Wu Chi you feel naturally comfortable. It is your neutral posture, your position of origin. All other positions can simply be regarded as a displacement from this.

Here, we delicately exploit the position of origin. By making slight variations from the centre, here and there, we come to understand Wu Chi and, consequently, ourselves at a deeper level. Deviations from the centre let us understand 'neutral' better.

Our standing posture can be seen as a bell with a striking pendulum inside. Our body is the bell, and our centre is the pendulum. As the bell tilts or moves, the pendulum adjusts itself accordingly.

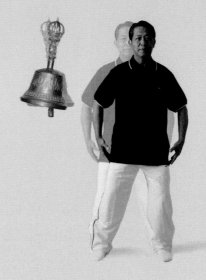

Above Starting in the neutral Wu Chi position, shift your weight slightly to the left so that it is distributed 60 per cent in the left leg and 40 per cent in the right leg. Feel your centre realign itself. Now try this with the other side.

> **Please note** *For the following two postures, it is strongly recommended that you spend less time on the forward-tilting Wu Chi posture, as it is less suitable for people with high blood pressure or heart problems.*

1 From neutral, shift 60 per cent of your weight to your heels, 40 per cent to the front of your feet. Again, you should feel the realignment of your centre.

2 From the neutral position shift your weight slightly, giving 60 per cent of your weight to the front of your feet, 40 per cent to the heels.

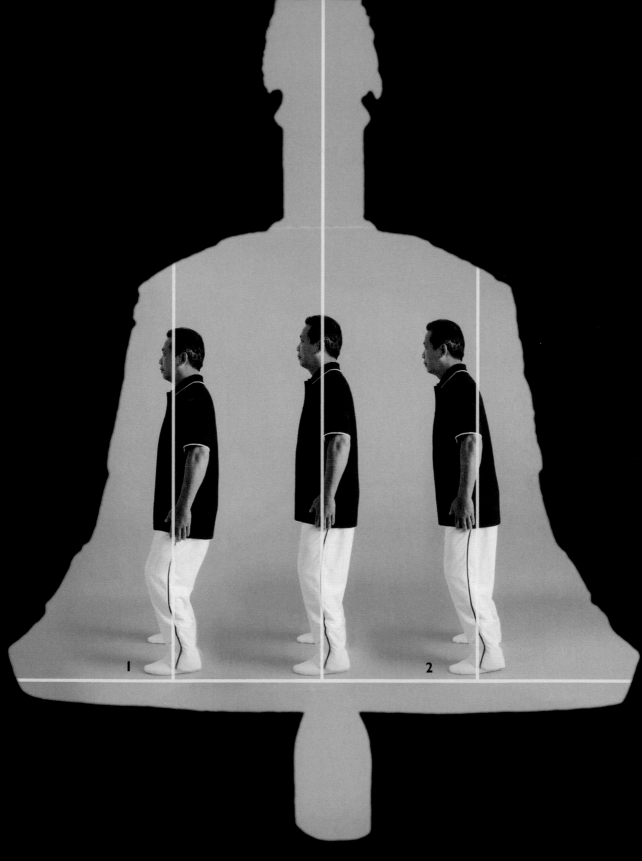

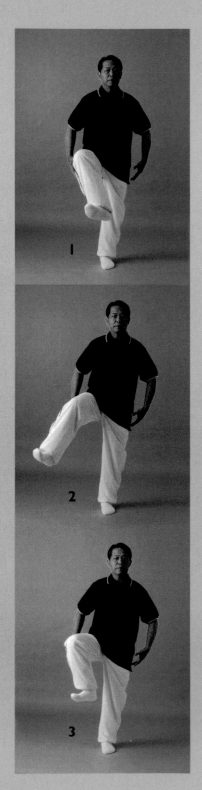

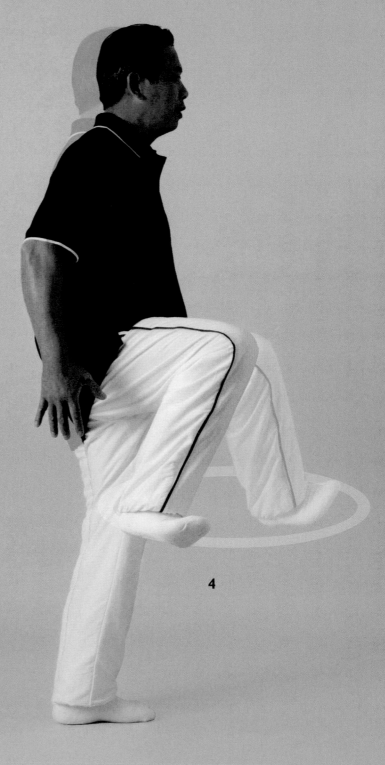

Circling your feet

This exercise trains both legs at the same time, each in a different manner. It is as if two dissimilar pieces of a jigsaw, from different places, are joined together agreeably.

For one leg, the training is heavy and grave. There are no external movements; everything is internal and unseen. The leg supporting your entire weight builds up strength and endurance. For the other leg, the training is light and carefree. The workout is purely external, based on active movement. This leg develops flexibility and elasticity.

Overall, this exercise develops coordination and balance. You balance on only one leg while the other leg moves. This practice not only develops knee flexibility and leg strength, it also, more subtly, works your hips and pelvic region, which connect your torso to your feet.

If you find standing on one leg too challenging, support yourself with a chair by your side. When you are circling your right foot, place the chair by your left, and vice versa.

In the beginning, circle each foot ten times. As you progress, increase to 30 times. You need not circle your foot quickly, however, since speed is not the priority here; a steady slow pace of rotation is more important.

1 Stand upright with your head forward and your right leg raised. Your arms curve naturally down from your shoulders, and your palms face your thighs. Keep your right knee still and flex your right ankle bringing the foot back slightly.

2 Circle your right foot clockwise while keeping your knee parallel with the floor and your thigh still.

3 Your right foot should remain flexed throughout. Only the lower right leg moves, the rest of your body should remain still.

4 From this side view, you can see that your supporting left leg should not be locked straight. Your thigh is kept horizontal and your knee hardly moves.

After circling your right foot, start again with your left. Raise your left knee and begin circling counterclockwise.

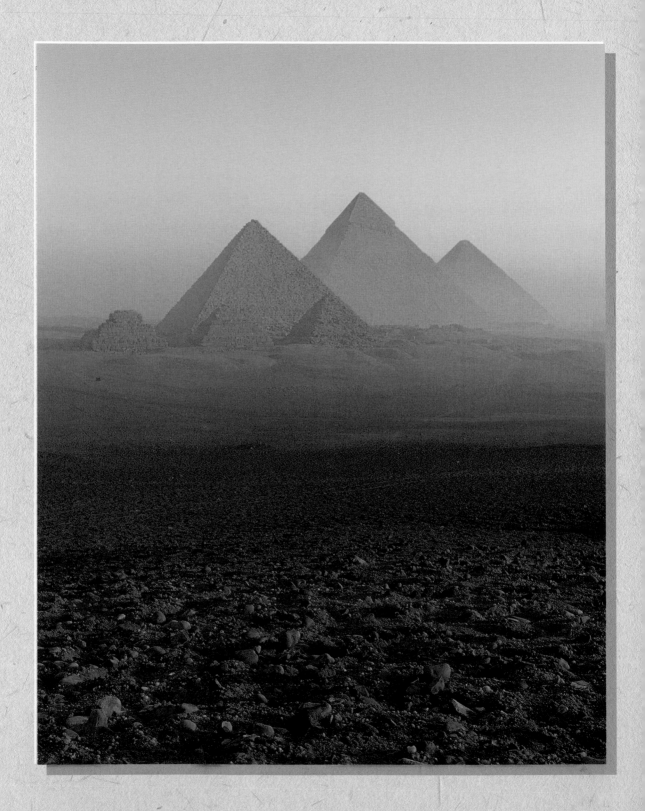

PART THREE

THE SIX DIRECTIONAL FORCES

Tao gives birth to One,
One gives birth to Two,
Two gives birth to Three,
Three gives birth to Myriad Things.

LAO TSE

The quotation above, is an extract from *Tao Te Ching* written by, probably, the greatest sage of ancient China, Lao Tse. Although open to many interpretations, it expresses brilliantly the evolution of existence out of nothingness. It numerically reveals the transformation of nullity into infinity. This intriguing concept is one of the founding pillars of Eastern philosophy, and is manifested in many places. In this chapter, you will see a subtle example.

Zhan Zhuang, the marvellous system of internal energy exercises, is a stationary and motionless art. Its stillness, and apparent absence of movements, demonstrate that your external appearance is irrelevant and, after a fashion, illusory. You are like a point with no breadth, width, or length. You are without dimension.

Your centre, the Tan Tien, is also a dimensionless, invisible point. Your force and inner strength are equally intangible. In Zhan Zhuang you are operating within a world of zero dimension.

Walking is, however, an entirely different matter. It is a form of travelling, taking you from one place to another, and one point to another. In our reality, mobility has three different dimensions.

The transition from standing to walking Chi Kung is a transition from emptiness to existence, from nothing to something. A point that previously had no dimension becomes active in three dimensions. You have gained a presence in the spatial realm and become dimensional.

This spatial evolution is one manifestation of Lao Tse's teachings, some 2,500 years ago. However, it cannot be achieved without hard work and training. To gain volume, you need to work on the three underlying axes. With two directions on each axis, there are six fundamental directions on which you need to focus. That is the aim and theme of this particular chapter: the six directional forces.

With the six directions, your centre will become like a point sandwiched between the bases of two pyramids, one above and one upside-down below. Your centre can travel linearly to each of the six corners – two peak corners and four, shared, base corners. This shape outlines the basic movability of your centre point. It, in turn, is the foundation of spatial mobility and movement.

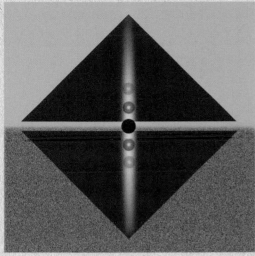

Your centre point can travel in two directions vertically…

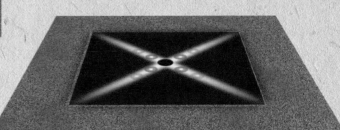

…and in four directions laterally…

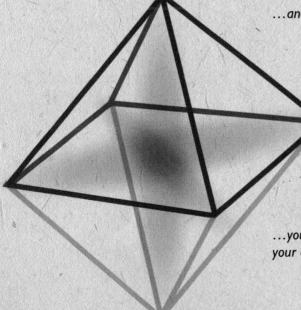

…you have the potential to move your centre in six directions.

Up and down

Let us begin our dimensional transformation with the vertical axis; the one that makes us special in the animal kingdom; the axis that defines us — standing. In some ways, it may be our most important dimension. How often do we instinctively equate strength with stature and height?

To begin this exercise you have to start with Wu Chi, the neutral position. Its intricate posture is already outlined in the previous chapter (see pages 56–57). Here, the aim is to move your centre up and down to gain dimension; you do so by moving your body up and down.

There should be no movements above your waist. Your arms, head, and torso should remain perfectly still. When you sink your centre down, bend only your knees. Exhale slowly and calmly as your height lowers. As you raise your centre, straighten your legs and inhale deeply but naturally.

Apart from the obvious leg training, this exercise also works the waist and pelvic region. Though this is subtle, it is also very important.

Initially, practise this 'up and down' movement slowly ten times. As you improve, build up gradually to 30 repetitions.

Please note *As you become familiar with the movement, let it adapt to the rhythm of your breath. Your breathing should dictate the pace of your movement and not the other way around. Perform natural breathing.*

I Move your centre up and down at an even pace. Let the movements become a rhythm in your mind. Your legs must not be fully straightened or locked in a vertical alignment at any time. Do not bend your legs too much — your knees should never protrude further than your toes. This limitation means that your knees bend and straighten only moderately during this exercise routine.

2 In this exercise, your legs have an underlying structure and elasticity. You are not simply sinking your weight by bending your knees. Imagine that there are two strong vertical springs fixed between your hips and ankles. As you move up, it takes effort to stretch the springs taut. As you relax, the springs pull you back down. Oscillate between stretching and loosening the springs, and keep your body as relaxed as possible.

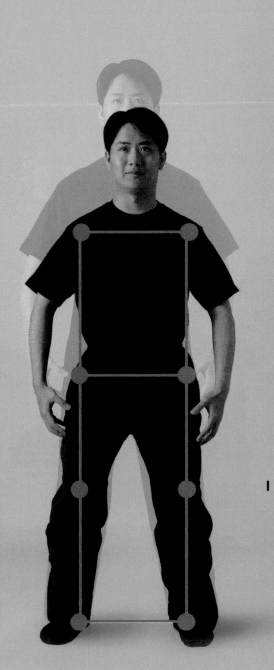

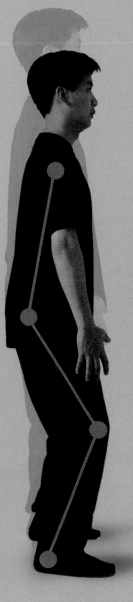

1

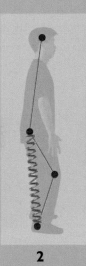

2

Left and right

The training exercise for movement along your second axis involves the arms. Here, your centre shifts to the right and left horizontally. The overall coordination in this workout is more complicated than the previous exercise, Up and Down.

In this particular exercise, the loose movements make it seem carefree and easy. Indeed, the movement is meant to be comfortable and relaxing, but it is not as simple as it appears. Beneath the surface, is a complicated system of puppets and puppeteers orchestrating the movements.

Each arm is raised to the side, one at a time, in a soft and gentle gesture. It is as if there is a string tied to your wrist pulling it up from above. When lifted, the arm remains loose and the elbow hangs down; the shoulder is not raised or stiffened; there is no strength in the arm; and the hand is equally relaxed with the fingers apart and curved. You are like a puppet with an invisible puppeteer pulling your strings.

As one of your arms is raised to the side, your body and your centre also move to that side. Imagine there is an elastic string attached between your wrist and your hip. The hip is also pulled as your arm moves out, but proportionally less far. Try to avoid tilting your body or sticking your hip out. The body, head, and other arm should remain relatively still; they simply shift horizontally. Your weight shifts with the distribution of 60 and 40 per cent. You are both the puppeteer and the puppet. You orchestrate your own movements by pulling your own strings.

Your breathing needs to be coordinated with your movements. As the arm is raised, inhale deeply. Exhale as it lowers again. Let yourself slowly attune to the rhythm of natural breathing.

Practise both sides, in alternating order, ten times. As you progress, increase gradually to 30 repetitions.

1 From the Wu Chi position (see pages 56–57), slowly lift your right wrist to the side to shoulder height, inhaling deeply and calmly. As you do this, slide your weight to the right so that 60 per cent is in the right leg and 40 per cent is in the left.

2 Lower your arm and exhale as you return to the neutral Wu Chi position. Your weight is once again evenly distributed between both legs. Pause briefly in Wu Chi before continuing.

Repeat the movement on the other side. Raise the left hand and shift your weight toward the left.

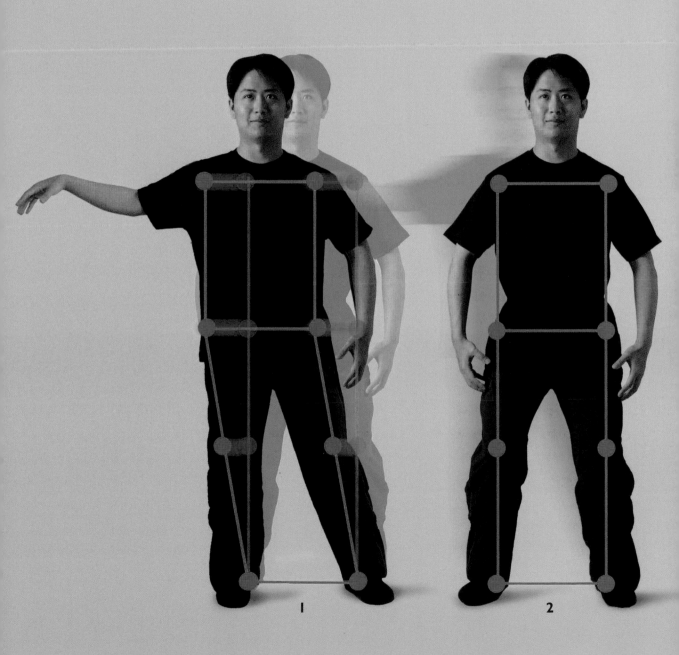

1

2

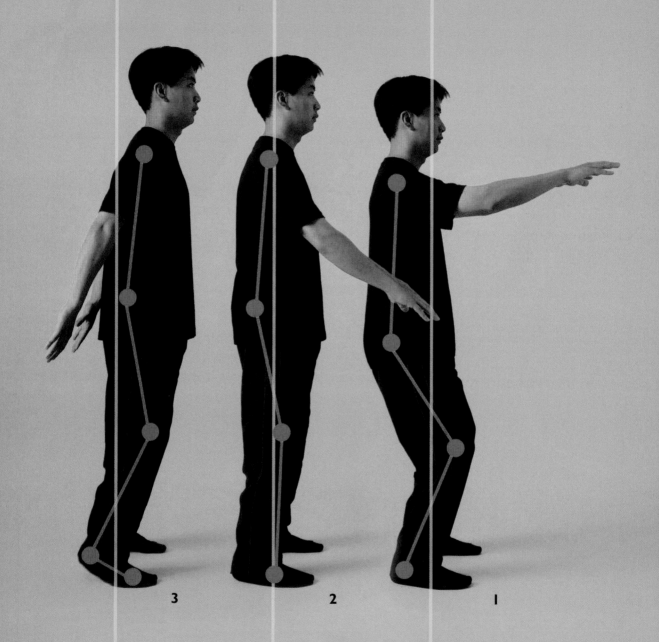

Forward and backward

Please note *Use your natural breathing rhythm to guide the pace of this exercise. Breathe in as your arms drop, and breathe out as you raise them.*

1 Stand in Wu Chi (see pages 56–57). Raise both your arms in front of you, palms down. Move your body back slightly by sinking your weight a little, then move 60 per cent of your weight on to your heals. Your raised arms support your balance – your body should neither tilt forward nor backward.

2 Lower your arms gently as if they are stroking the air. At the same time, straighten your legs slightly. Your centre will move forward.

3 Gently swing your hands back behind you, letting the momentum bring your body forward. Do not stick out your chest or tilt your body forward. Bend your knees a little, lifting your heels very slightly off the ground, so that 60 per cent of your weight is now on the balls of your feet.

In the previous two exercises you were moving up and down, or left and right. Your centre was travelling vertically or horizontally with a good approximation to the true axes. However, this third axis is a little different and a lot more complicated. This is the hardest of the three-dimensional exercises described in this chapter.

Like all spatial objects, the human body has length, breadth, and width. Lengthways, we are more than adequate. We are relatively tall creatures in the animal kingdom, given our mass. The 'up and down' exercise involves only our legs, which can move our centre vertically over a considerable distance. In the 'left and right' exercise, our movement is restricted by the width of our body. In the Wu Chi posture (see pages 56–57), our centre has room to move horizontally, but considerably less than it could vertically.

The breadth of the human body, front to back, offers the greatest limitation. Unlike four-legged mammals, such as cats and dogs, we have very little front to back distance. What we have gained in height by standing, we have lost in breath. Given this limitation, the 'forward and backward' movement described here, does not move our centre, perfectly along this particular axis. The approximation is fairly crude in relation to the directional force of the other two exercises.

Initially, practise the movements ten times. In time, slowly increase to 30 times.

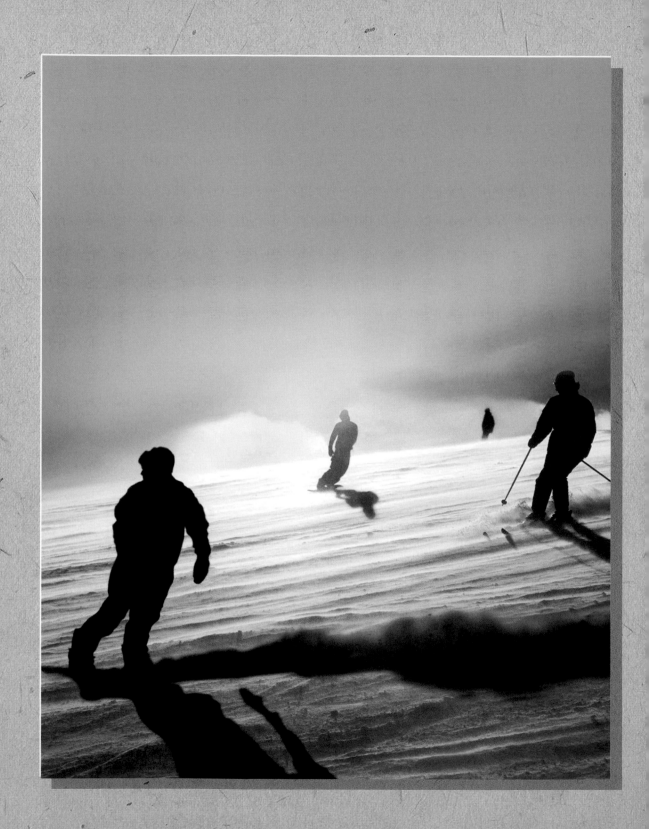

PART FOUR

KNOWING YOUR STEPS

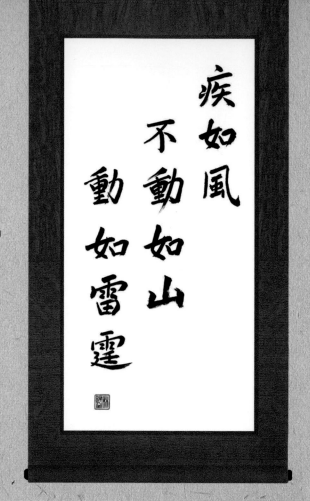

Swift as the Wind…
Motionless as the Mountain…
Move like the Thunder…

SUN TSE, CALLIGRAPHY (RIGHT) BY MASTER LAM

Here, we have a brilliant set of analogies regarding mobility, written by the prominent Sun Tse, probably the greatest strategist in ancient history. They refer to travelling in one of its most extreme forms, its application to violence. Though slightly tangential to our theme, these insightful statements on the extreme execution of mobility are nonetheless paramount. They give us a glimpse of the true essence of mobility.

However, the edge that travelling offers is double-sided. When you walk, you are transferring yourself from one place to another with your legs. It is a process of change, and change can be violent. It can be unsettling, and leave you vulnerable. Throughout the ages there has been much literature, studying, researching, and guiding you safely along this and other processes of change.

In the art of Da Cheng Chuan, where Zhan Zhuang is the stationary element, Tsou Pu is considered its mobile counterpart. The term, Tsou Pu, literally means 'running steps'. It is a system of leg exercises involving a variety of carefully executed walks. Contrary to its name, this branch of the art does not demand speed. Swiftness and momentum emerge from some of the movements, but only after much practice.

Tsou Pu is the 'leg' equivalent of Shih Li, the system of power training within Da Cheng Chuan that is practised mainly with the arms. It is these various associations, and its own unique structure, which makes Tsou Pu a system of its own.

Misleading though its name may be, the essence of Tsou Pu actually demands stability, balance, and flexibility. Indeed, it has the same requirement as when one is in a stationary position. This branch of Da Cheng Chuan draws on, and emphasizes, one apparently contradicting idea: stillness while in motion.

In Tsou Pu, you seek a state of inner stillness even when you are in motion. It is like trying to be a smooth, round ball. Any irregular shape would have various points of balance when resting on a flat surface, whereas, a round ball is always in a state of equilibrium, however it is laid, even when it is rolling. Your aim is to achieve this flexible, moving equilibrium.

The physics of objects in motion is, in some aspects, very different from the physics of stationary objects. This is seen in every-day life. A bike, which cannot balance when at rest, can remain upright when moving. Similarly, a bridge can support passing weight more readily than a resting load. This difference in dynamics and inner work is what gives Tsou Pu a spotlight of its own. This is also the reason why the practice of Tsou Pu is often reserved for intermediate and advanced students of Da Cheng Chuan, rather than for beginners.

SOME GENERAL GUIDANCE

The Tsou Pu exercises described in the following pages are a colourful inspiration. Each is unique, differing in appearance and spirituality. Do not be overwhelmed by the variety of movements within these pages. They come from a common source and share the same underlying structure.

Grand Master Wang Xiang Zhai, the founder of Da Cheng Chuan, offered much guidance to the practice of Tsou Pu. He explained how one needs to be like a cat when practising steps and walking systems. This deceptively simple analogy is a crystallization of vast knowledge and experience.

When a cat walks, it is with much pride and confidence. Cats are territorial creatures and know their own ground. Every step they take is full of familiarity and a sense of control. Their steps are also filled with ease. Their movements are relaxed and smooth.

Although cats are famous for appearing carefree, you should not associate this ease with carelessness or being off-guard. Agile and flexible while walking, cats are extremely quick to react to changing circumstances. Their sharpness is always there – it may be dormant, but is never absent. These collective feline virtues are the spirit behind the analogy. Try to emulate these qualities when practising the Tsou Pu exercises.

Another important piece of advice for practising the following steps, is to remember that your legs are an extension of your body. This can be more easily understood when looking at the arms. The arms, being also a pair of body extensions, do not dictate the movements of the body. They are submissive rather than assertive. Whenever the arms are out of reach, the body moves forward to offer the arms assistance. In terms of mobility, the hierarchy of control is naturally recognized, the body above and the arms below.

Your legs and feet, however, less readily recognize in this chain of command. Your feet directly influence your balance. For most people, their legs direct the movement of the body. Therefore, when your feet slip, you simply lose control and fall. Your body has carelessly given away authority to the legs.

This must be consciously avoided when practising Tsou Pu. Your body should manage the legs rather than the other way around. If the feet are out of reach, the body should then move to offer support. When your centre is in control, your chance of losing balance is greatly reduced. The authority should always return to your centre.

The Crane Steps

In Chinese culture, the white crane is a highly respected bird. In the past, the crane was even considered sacred. Cranes are creatures of longevity and are frequent companions of the Gods and Immortals in traditional legends. Over centuries, many artists and craftsmen have sought inspiration from this revered bird, and tried to reflect its essence in their works.

This source of inspiration is by no means restricted to fine and applied arts. Past Chinese masters of martial and physical arts, have also studied the crane. One folktale relates that it was from observing a fight between a snake and a crane that the legendary Zhang San Feng was inspired to found Tai Chi Chuan.

The movement described here, is another manifestation. It draws on the essence of the crane's style of walking. Unlike human legs, which bend backward, crane legs bend forward. Their walking gesture is, therefore, naturally intrusive.

When you practise this movement, it is important to emulate this intrusive attribute of the crane's walk. Your feet should step forward in a very direct and acute manner, but without any hint of hostility or aggression.

The characteristic walk of the crane is space-invasive, but neither challenging nor threatening. It walks in a very carefree and light-hearted fashion. Your practice should be equally subtle and relaxed.

In the beginning, your movement should be delicately slow, like a whisper in the night. When you feel that you have made much progress, pick up the pace slightly. You should aim to be proficient at this movement in slow motion, and at your natural pace. Practise slowly in order to learn all the minute intricacies of this exercise. Practise at normal speed to see how much you understand them.

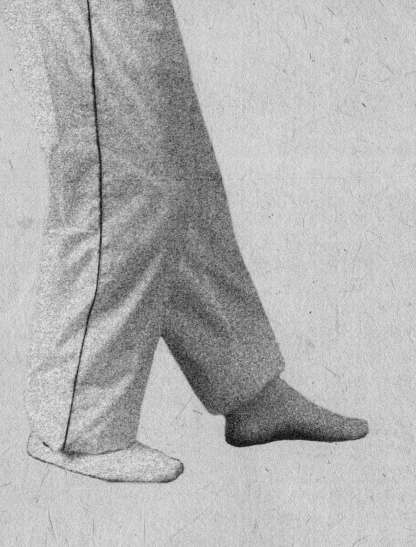

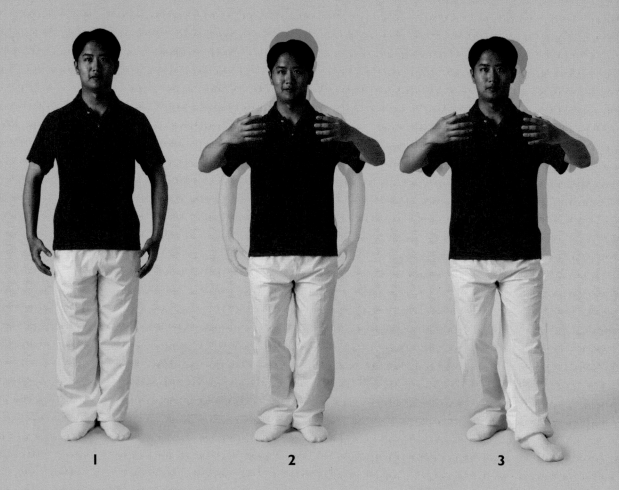

1   2   3

1 To begin, stand with your heels together and feet at 45 degrees. Stand straight and upright, but not in a stiff, military way. The shoulders, hips, and knees should all be loose and relaxed. Let your arms hang naturally from your shoulders, but remain subtly firm. Gaze forward and breathe calmly.

2 Raise both hands up in front of you to shoulder-level. Bend your knees and sink your weight a little. Avoid stiffening the shoulders, and avoid having your elbows stick out too much to the sides. Imagine you are holding a huge balloon and your arms are wrapping around it almost entirely. Keep your fingers straight and slightly apart.

3 Without moving your upper body, extend your left foot outward. Keep your weight mostly in your right leg. Do not lift the left foot too high; it should appear as if it is touching the ground through-out the movement. Glide it forward in a smooth and gentle fashion. This emulates the essence of the crane's forward-bending legs. Although fully extended, do not let your left leg become locked straight.

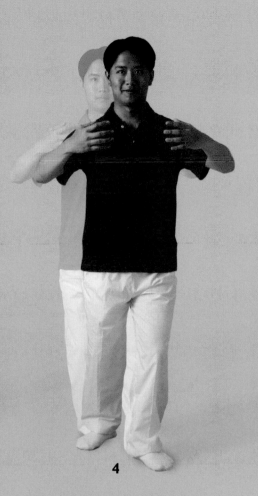

4

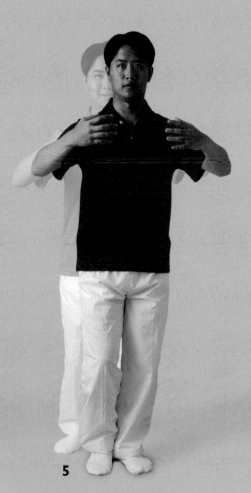

5

4 Press your right foot against the ground to straighten the leg. Glide your upper body forward toward your left foot, shifting your weight as you do so. Do not turn your body or your gaze by very much, and keep your upper body at the same level throughout.

5 As you balance yourself with your forward leg, draw your back leg up from behind. Step your right foot forward, keeping it close to the ground. Your heels touch, once again, but the right heel should be slightly raised.

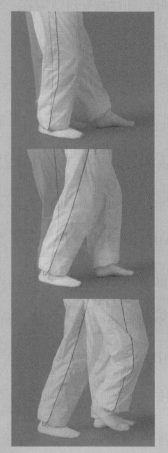

Left *From the side, you can see more clearly how these steps are made. Simply by straightening the left leg, the left foot automatically takes a small, smooth step forward. This means that the stride is rather short, and it is taken in a light and casual manner.*

Overall, this exercise is very subtle, and its pace should be equally light and carefree.

Variation *You may choose to turn your body slightly to the right and face in the direction that the right foot is pointing. Whether you decide to turn the body or not, just remember to stick to the same decision throughout the practice. The turning of the waist is illustrated in steps 7, 8 and 9.*

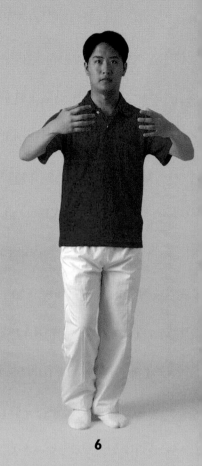

6

6 Pause for a moment and notice that your two legs are held differently; your left leg is bent slightly, while your right leg is bent slightly more. This small difference is significant.

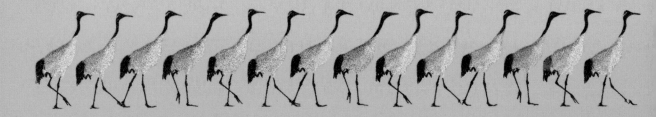

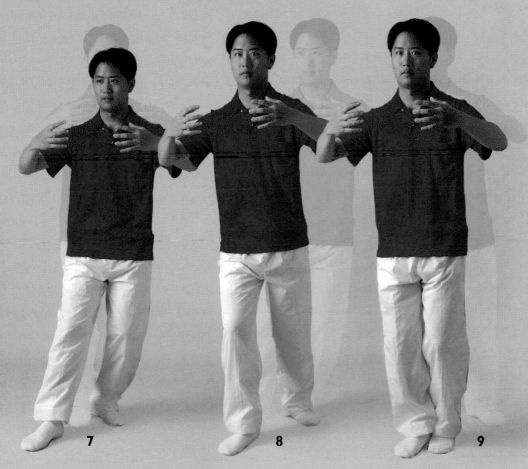

7 Take a small step forward and slightly towards the right with your right foot. Keep all your weight on your left leg, leaving your right leg light and flexible.

8 Extend your left leg and bend your right knee. Gently glide your body forward as you shift your weight from one leg to the other. Avoid tilting your body.

9 As you secure your weight and balance entirely on the right leg, bring your left foot forward. Your heels touch, once again, although the left heel is slightly raised. From here, go to Step 3 to continue the walk.

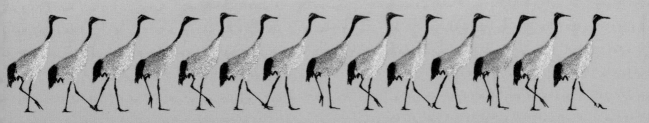

Mo Ca ~ The Ice Steps

The Chinese name for this step (pronounced Mo Cha) conveys the idea of friction and erosion, thus reflecting its inner meaning. Its alternative name – one with a more Western tone – is The Ice Step. This term also reflects an important underlying element in this movement.

It is, essentially, a step movement with a questioning attribute. Throughout this sequence, imagine yourself on the surface of a frozen lake. You are cautious and alert as you step, lest you crack the ice. Your feet do not simply move forward; they carefully explore as they advance. In each and every centimetre of progress, you are preparing for the unpredictable; your foot is like an adventurer in unknown territory. You test the ice for strength before giving weight to the foot yet, even then, the weight is cautiously given.

Another way to understand this exercise is to imagine that you are a fire-fighter in a smoke-filled room; your steps are part of your sight, your only visibility is sensation.

You should only raise your feet infinitesimally. From an observer's perspective you appear not to have lifted them at all. It is as if you are wearing skis. Your feet simply move along the surface of the floor. Hence, the Chinese name for this particular movement.

Throughout this sequence, alertness and caution should radiate from you. However, this should not convey stress or tension. Your mind should remain relaxed, and your heart light. Try to avoid feeling anxious. Your movements must be firm and steady, but not hard or rigid.

Do not mistake caution for anxiety, or confuse firmness with stiffness. It may be a thin line, physically and mentally, but it makes a world of difference.

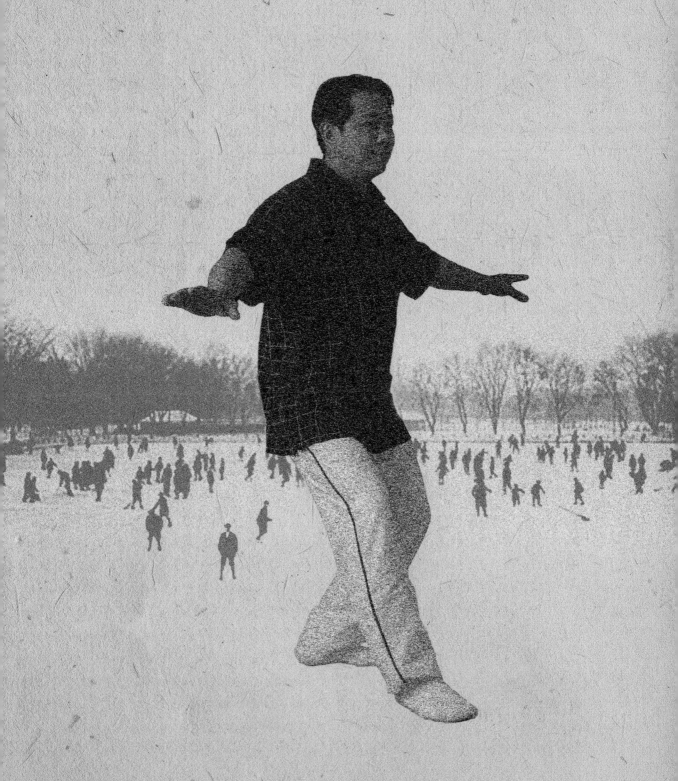

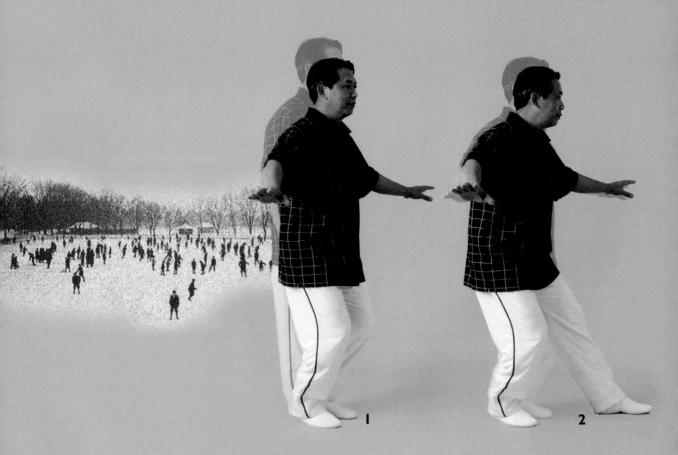

1 Stand in Wu Chi (see pages 56–57). Breathe slowly and deeply until your mind is calm. Raise your hands to the sides and bend both knees moderately. Your hands rest, palms down, at the same level as your waist. Your shoulders remain relaxed. It is as if you are half-submerged in water with your hands floating on the surface.

2 Imagine the floor is made of ice. Sink your weight into your right leg and carefully slide your left foot forward, tracing an arc across the surface of the floor. Your foot should be light and weightless, offering no pressure to the ground. Try not to confuse the feeling of caution with stalling stagnation. At the same time, turn your waist so that your body and gaze move left. Keep your upper body, arms, and head relatively still.

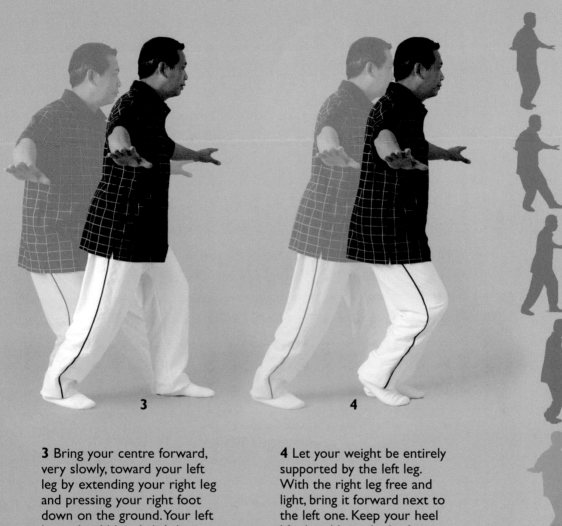

3 Bring your centre forward, very slowly, toward your left leg by extending your right leg and pressing your right foot down on the ground. Your left knee should bend slightly. There is no movement above the waist, and your centre should remain at the same level throughout the move.

4 Let your weight be entirely supported by the left leg. With the right leg free and light, bring it forward next to the left one. Keep your heel lifted, and let only the front of your right foot touch the ground. Both legs are bent; the right leg slightly more than the left.

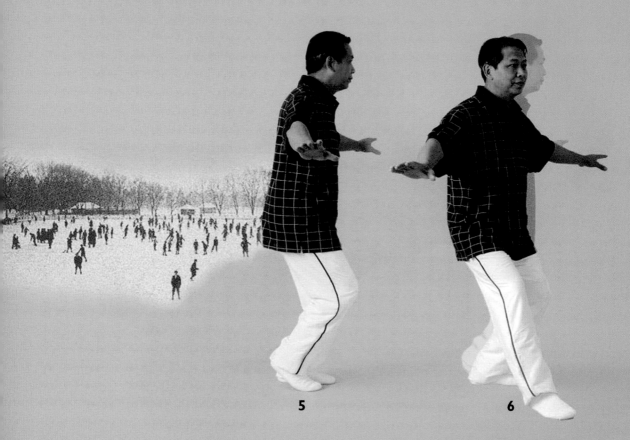

5

6

5 Having completed the first part of the sequence you must now prepare for the next. Pause and make sure all your weight is on your left foot.

6 Circle your right foot out and to the right, clockwise. Turn both your gaze and your body in that direction. As your foot stretches forward in the arc, lower the heel – keep your weight in your left foot. Although you have rotated your body, everything above your waist remains relatively still, and your centre stays unchanged. Notice that your right knee is still very slightly bent.

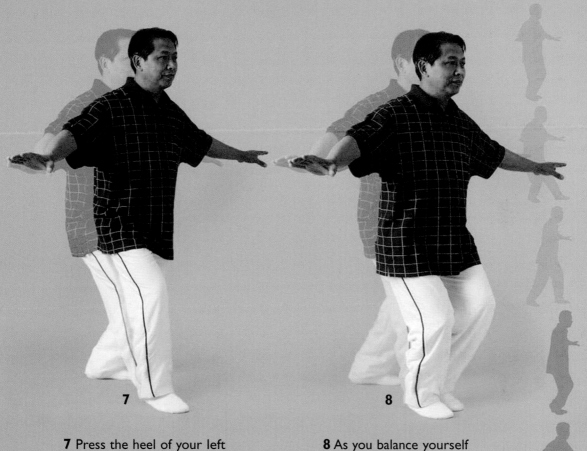

7

8

7 Press the heel of your left foot against the ground to straighten the leg. Bend your right leg at the same time. Little by little you are transferring your weight from one leg to the other, slowly moving your body forward. Remember to keep your upper body at the same level throughout.

8 As you balance yourself entirely on your right leg, bring your left one forward. Your feet touch each other, but the left heel is raised. Your knees are both slightly bent – your left leg more so than your right. From here, proceed to step 2 and repeat the sequence.

The 'Spading' Steps

Unlike the other exercises in this section, this sequence
involves a great deal of waist movement and tilting of the
upper body. Because of this, the bearing and body coordination here may appear quite confusing and complicated.
However, knowing the source of its inspiration can provide
insight to the essence and practice of the exercise.

The source of inspiration goes back to one of the
earliest activities of human civilization – farming. As farming
is so much a part of world culture, it is no surprise that many
colourful traditions and inspirations come from this source.
The step movement described here, mimics the action of a
farmer digging and loosening his soil.

As the farmer digs his spade into the soil, he leans
forward onto his front leg. This is refined and formalized into
the bending and shifting of the body in this sequence. Then, as
the farmer lifts the load on his spade, he straightens up. Bear
this image in mind when you practise this sequence. It will
aid your coordination and alignment.

Notice that the arms are relatively motionless. All
movements come from the waist and below. This is very
important. When digging, the main strength does not come
from the arms, as you might assume. It comes upward from
the legs, but this does not mean that the arms can become
lifeless. Their role is simply different from what you might
expect. The arms act as levers and supports. They are complementary tools that aid the movements of the legs.

Given the complex body coordination required to
compete The 'Spading' Step, it is important to practise it
slowly at first. This will make it easier for you to understand
its various intricacies and help you avoid being overwhelmed
by the wave-like motion.

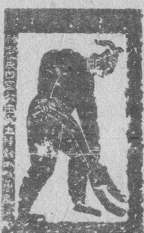

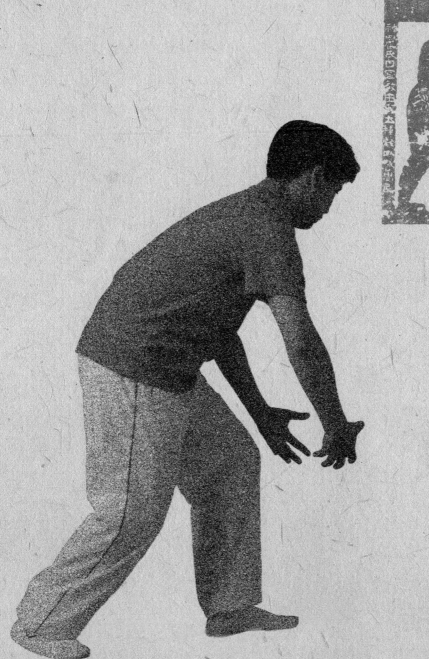

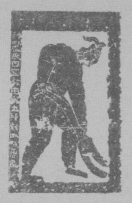

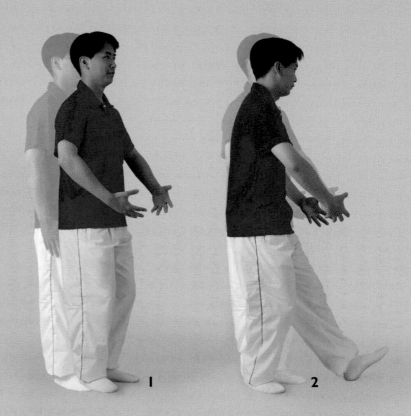

1 Stand comfortably upright with your heels together and your arms hanging naturally, elbows slightly bent. Lift both hands in front of you to the level of your belly. Curve your arms and hands as if you are holding a large ball in front of you. At the same time, sink your weight slightly, bending your knees.

2 In one smooth motion, turn your gaze and your body slightly to your left, and take a small step in that direction with your left foot, so that it stretches out in a curve. Place your left heel down, but keep your toes raised. Avoid pulling your toes too far back or straightening your left leg entirely. Your weight rests mainly on your right leg.

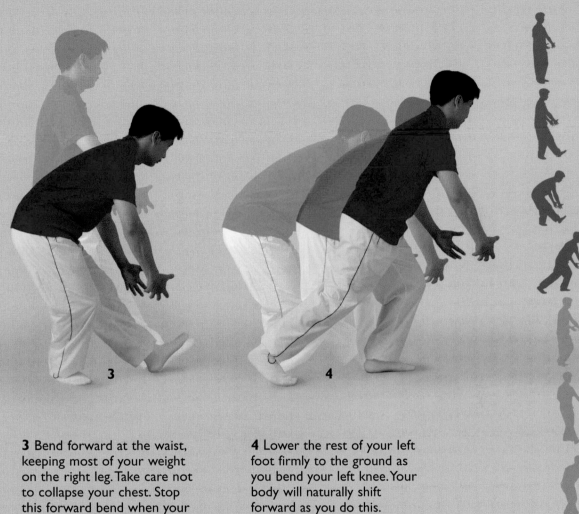

3 Bend forward at the waist, keeping most of your weight on the right leg. Take care not to collapse your chest. Stop this forward bend when your hands are approximately level with your knees. Do not look down, but look ahead.

4 Lower the rest of your left foot firmly to the ground as you bend your left knee. Your body will naturally shift forward as you do this.

Press down into the ground with the front of your right foot, straightening your leg moderately. Lift your right heel slightly, and slowly begin to straighten your body.

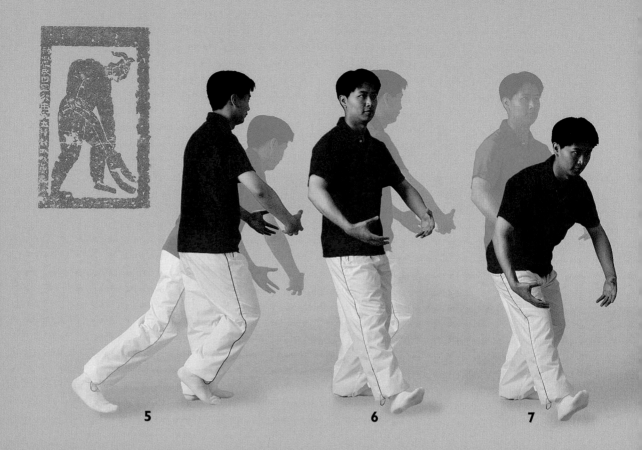

5 Bring your body back to the upright position by drawing your right foot forward. As your body straightens, your hands are once again in front of your belly. Your left leg is almost straight with the foot flat on the ground, while your right leg is slightly bent with the heel raised.

6 Keeping most of your weight in your left leg, in one smooth motion, circle your right foot out to the right, turning your body in that direction as you do so. Place your right heel gently on the ground, bending your left leg accordingly.

7 Bend at the waist without shifting your weight forward. Your head, body, and arms should be relatively still. Sink your weight slightly by bending your left leg.

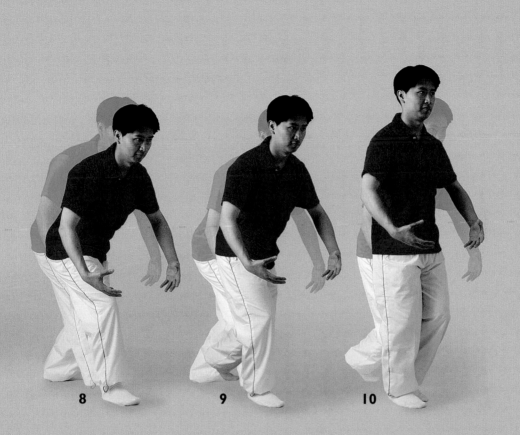

8 Lower your right foot completely, and bend the right knee slightly. Your body will shift forward and your weight will be more or less evenly distributed between both legs.

9 Press diagonally down with the ball of your left foot and raise the heel. Begin making yourself upright by straightening both legs.

10 Bring your left foot forward to rest beside your right foot. Your right leg becomes almost straight. Your right foot is flat on the ground while only the ball of your left foot touches the ground. This is the mirror image of step 5. From here, proceed to step 3 and repeat the entire sequence.

The Bear Steps

This exercise is yet another step movement that draws its name and inspiration from the animal kingdom. In appearance, it is probably the most simple step movement in this book but, actually, it is one of the more advanced practices. It is a demanding sequence usually reserved for the latter stages of Chi Kung training.

This powerful step portrays the essence of a bear during that brief moment when it stands upright on its hind legs. Your arms are raised with the palms facing out, fingers apart, emulating the claws of the bear. It is an outward intimidating gesture. This is a very direct and potent exercise.

The power, however, is not volatile. It is neither explosive nor ferocious. You are not like a bomb, bursting into energy, nor an inferno, blazing out your power.

Your strength is inert and, to some degree, stationary. You become a towering body of strength, just like the bear. Immense inner strength reveals itself but is by no means seeping out.

You advance forward, 2–5 cm (1–2 in) with each step. The movement may seem sluggish and your progress slow. Some of you may even feel vulnerable. However, that could not be further from the truth. You are more like a military tank, a slow but unstoppable force. You press onward gradually and inevitably.

Also, power should not be confused with aggression. The movement may be intimidating, but it is mild in its own way. Aggression is violence and anger; it leads to ferocity and offers no peace of mind. Remember, a bear can be as gentle as it is dangerous. When a bear stands, it does not inevitably attack. It is simply displaying strength and authority.

Because this particular sequence offers only minute movements, you may be tempted to concentrate too much on the posture and become tense. Try not to do this.

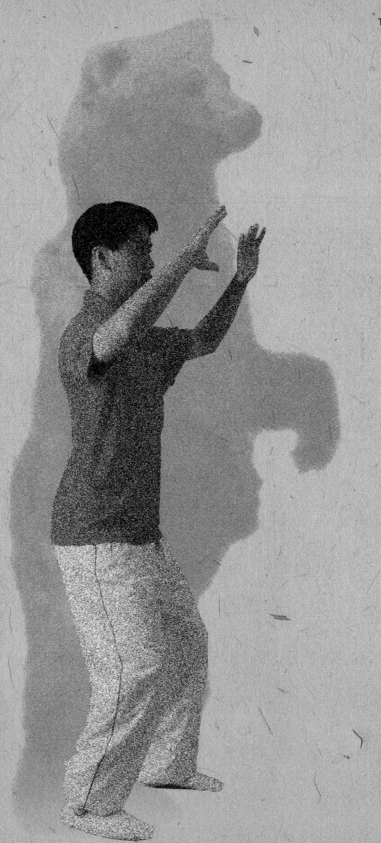

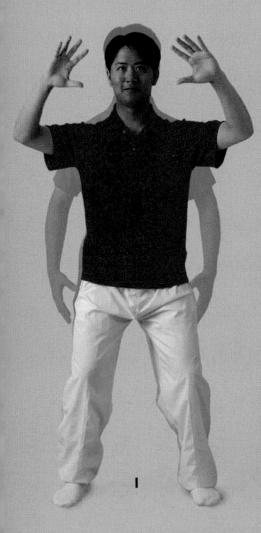

1

Please note *You should start the exercise from a relaxed standing posture. This is very similar to Wu Chi (see pages 56–57), but your feet are slightly further apart and your centre is lower. As you become more proficient in Wu Chi, you will feel how these minor changes, make a considerable difference.*

1 Raise both arms in front of you and turn your palms outward, level with your face, shoulder-width apart. Be careful not to have your legs too bent. Your knees should not stick out too far (see pages 48–49). Keep your arms relaxed but firm – it is as if you are pushing or pressing against a large balloon in front of you. Let your inner strength radiate from you as you stand in this posture. Make sure your weight is evenly distributed between both legs. Breathe slowly and deeply to clear your mind. Only when you feel calm should you begin the steps.

2 In this side view, you can see clearly how upright and intimidating is this posture. Just because your arms are raised in front of you, do not tilt your body. The movements in this exercise are so minute that they can barely be seen.

3 Take a small step of about 2–5 cm (1–2 in); making sure your feet remain parallel, pointing forward. Your weight should remain evenly distributed between both legs at all times. This is extremely important, as it distinguishes this step movement from all of the others. Do not shift your weight onto one leg in order to lift the other one.

The centre line of your body should not move laterally, aim to keep it as stable as possible. Take care not to move your body to the left or right at any time. Imagine you are pushing a huge ball forward, centimetre by centimetre.

You should only take a step with the other foot when you feel ready. Speed is of little importance, and each step should be made in one smooth movement.

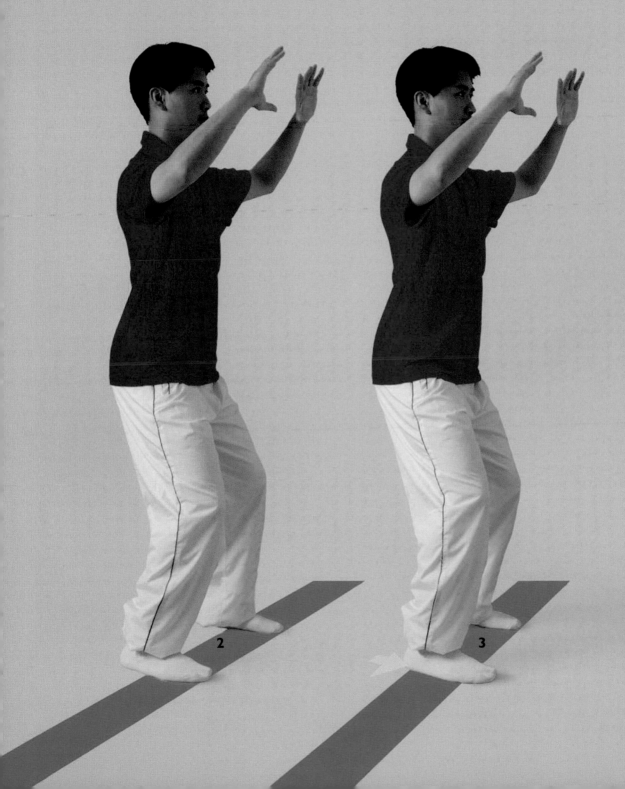

The Side Steps

This exercise differs from the others in this section in one important feature. The previous exercises took you forward, while this sequence takes you sideways.

There is no real walking here, in that you are not going anywhere. It is a form of stationary walking where you remain on the same spot throughout. As such, it is the most space-efficient of all the step exercises in this section. You can practise this almost anywhere.

Though the movements in this exercise are mainly leg movements, with the arms relatively stationary, it is important not to neglect the upper body. If you remember the last time you played tug-of-war, your hands clutched the rope as you heaved your body backward. Your arms and everything above the waist were stationary. You only moved your legs.

Here, the situation is similar. Although there are no movements in the arms or torso, they are by no means slack or limp. The tightness and inert strength of the arms is present, especially at the moment when you draw your body back. Your arms should radiate power downward from your hands, as though you are firing two rockets into the ground. Imagine you are pressing something down with your hands and keeping it under control. However, there is no tension, only inert strength. Your whole body should remain calm and relaxed throughout the exercise.

The inner sides of your thighs are also subtly trained here. As the legs are drawn together, the thighs are squeezed inward slightly. You may find it helpful to imagine that you are holding something, such as a large balloon, between your thighs. As the legs are pulled together, you squeeze the balloon lightly.

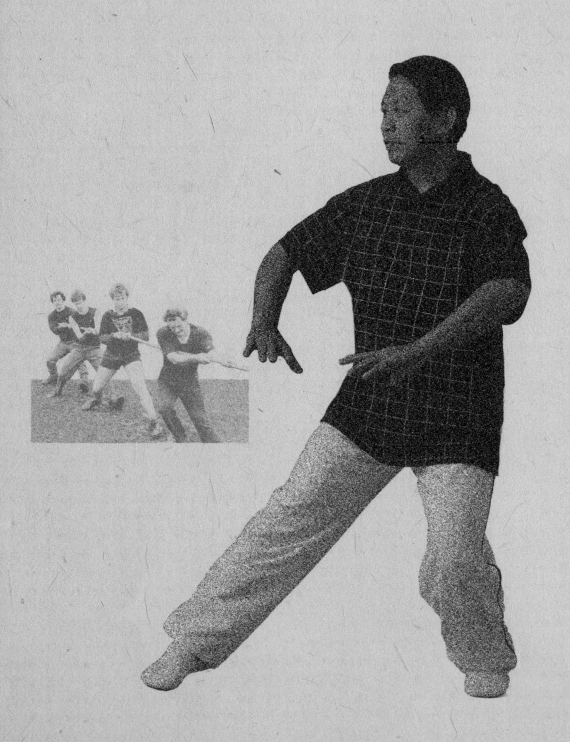

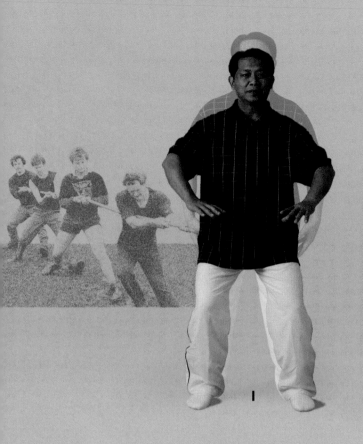

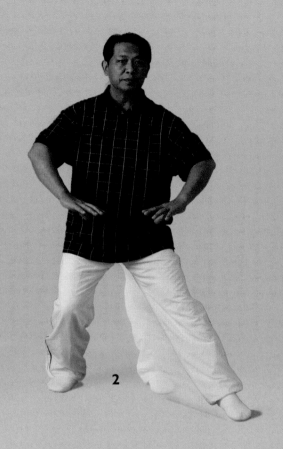

1 To begin, stand in Wu Chi (see pages 56–57). Bring your hands in front of you so they are level with your belly. Your palms are facing down. Bend your knees slightly to lower your weight. Your hands should be shoulder-width apart; the fingers separated and slightly curved. Turn both hands inward slightly so that the elbows are mildly raised. Do not have them stick out too far to the sides.

2 Stretch your left foot out to the left and straighten your left leg almost entirely. To do this, lift and then plant your left foot securely on the ground, making contact with your toes, but keeping the heel light and flexible. Have your left foot point forward. Your upper body and centre should not have moved. In order to keep your balance, your this side step needs to be swift and smooth.

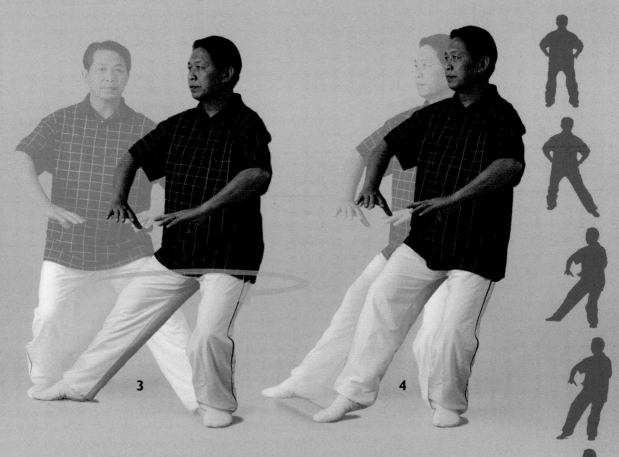

3 Swap the roles of your two legs by straightening one and bending the other – your left knee is bent and your right leg is nearly straight. Turn your right foot and your upper body clockwise, shifting your weight far to the left. Everything above the waist, your body, arms, and head, should remain relatively unchanged.

4 With your weight entirely on your left leg, gently draw your right foot back, raising the heel a little. Reduce the distance between your feet until it is, once again, approximately shoulder-width. The front of your right foot gently touches the ground throughout this withdrawal. Now, repeat the movements, but this time starting on the other side. Take a large side step with your right foot and let the toes point forward once again. This is a mirror image of step 2.

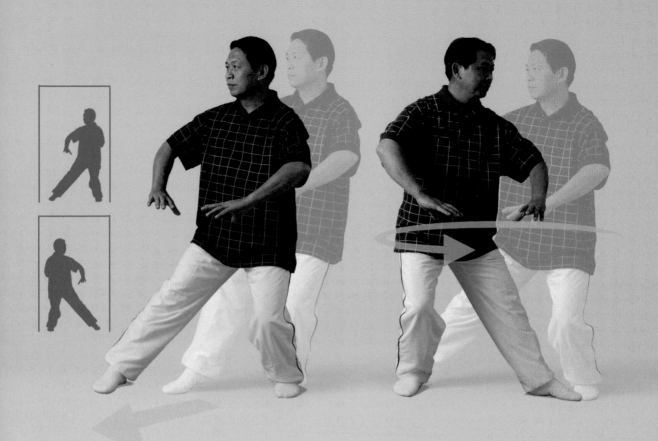

Please note As a whole, your movements in The Side Steps sequence should imitate a sliding door, opening and closing. Imagine that your upper body is the door; your legs and feet are the rails and tracks. Your centre is oscillating left and right throughout the exercise, as dictated by your leg positions. Overall, the level of body coordination needs to be good otherwise the door will not operate smoothly.

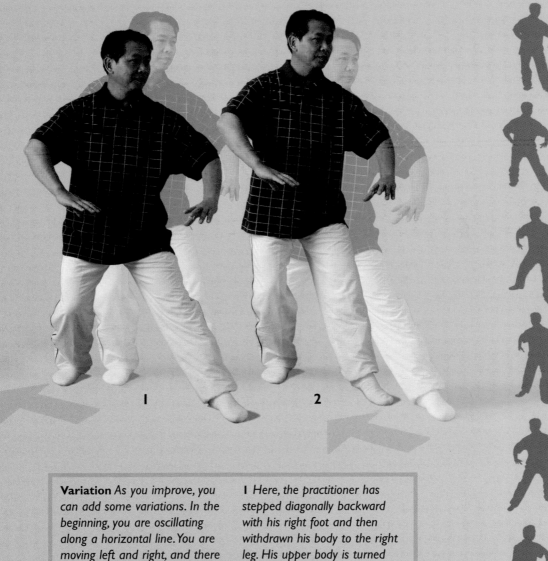

1

2

Variation As you improve, you can add some variations. In the beginning, you are oscillating along a horizontal line. You are moving left and right, and there is hardly any forward movement. However, this restriction is unnecessary for the more advanced practitioner. Rather than taking a lateral step, you can take a diagonal one. Both feet can step out diagonally forward or backward.

1 Here, the practitioner has stepped diagonally backward with his right foot and then withdrawn his body to the right leg. His upper body is turned slightly to the left.

2 Next, he pulls back the left foot toward his right foot, until they are shoulder-width apart.

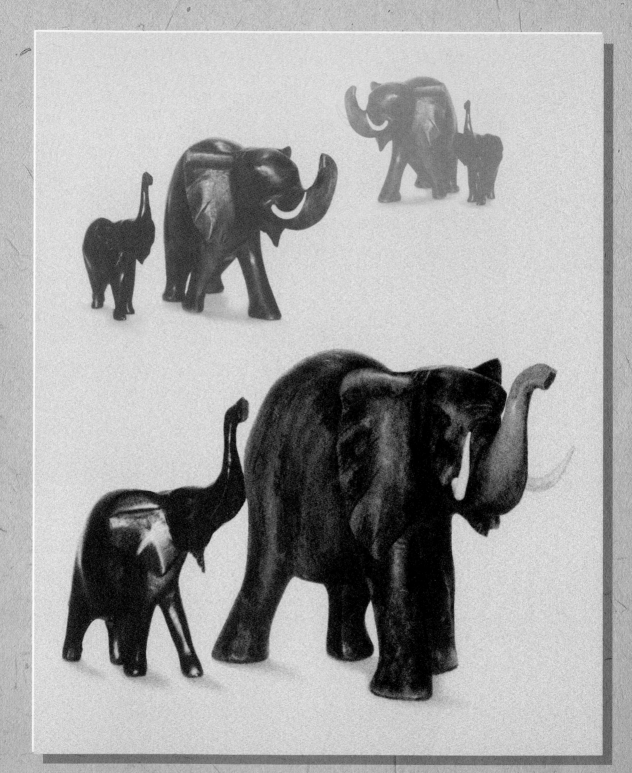

PART FIVE

THE WALKING SPECTRUM

We have already suggested earlier that strength does not come from the arms; it comes upward from the legs. The underlying meaning of this statement is profound. We have established the importance of the legs as daily carriers of our weight, as second hearts, and as reflections of our health (see page 55). However, the legs are also part of something greater, more elemental.

If we broaden our vision, we no longer see legs as simply limbs. We can see them as bridges. As the human body can be entirely expressed as a point, a nucleus within the body, your legs can be viewed as bridges that connect your centre to the Earth. This vital connection has immense significance.

Across the various lands and cultures of which this world is abundantly composed, creation myths share some similarities. One common theme is the idea that mankind is created from the Earth, and at the end of physical life, the body once again returns to the Earth. We live on the Earth and eat the fruits of the Earth. It is, therefore, no mere metaphor to say that we are children of the Earth. From this perspective, we can see more clearly that our legs are a parental connection to the Earth.

The connection is not merely a remnant of the mythical past; the bond is alive and vividly active. Consider the relation of fish to water. They are, in their own manifestations, children of water, as people are of land. If you are familiar with fishing, you will know that fish are creatures of considerable strength and speed, despite their size. However, such power and energy are lost as soon as they are out of water. They become weak and helpless. Their source of strength comes from being in the water.

This access to strength is true for us also. Our legs are like umbilical cords connecting us to the Mother Earth. Through them, strength and energy are drawn and exerted according to our will. If we are uprooted from the ground, as fish out of water, we become weak and helpless. Our true source of strength comes from our connection to the earth. When detached from it, we are vulnerable. It is, therefore, important to fortify the bond and establish a more potent connection. The following exercises specifi-cally fulfil that objective.

Each step sequence in this part of the book is complete and self-contained. They have been carefully selected from the many walking systems practised in China. They have various roots. By understanding their origins, you can gain greater insight and enrich your practice. These walking systems are the fruitions of much study, research, and experience from numerous past masters.

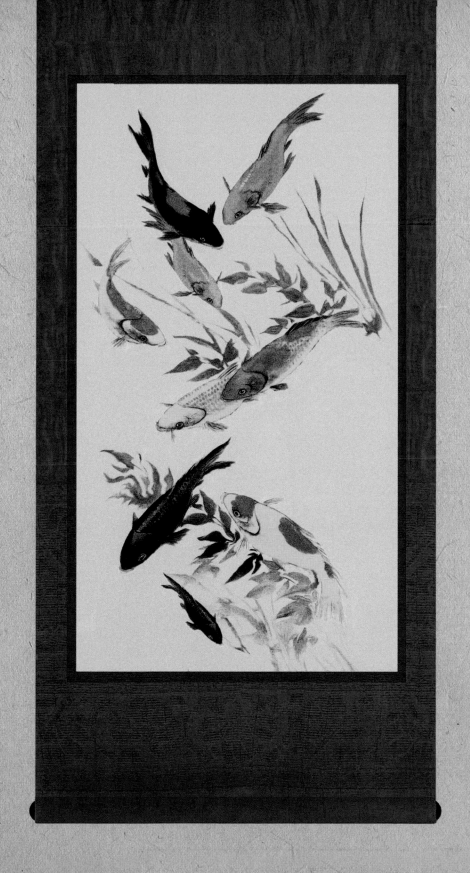

Reverse Walking of the Immortals

Travelling in reverse may be a strange and unnatural sight. People do not normally walk backward. The only time they do so is in moments of fright and, even then, they only take a few steps back.

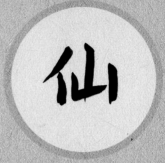

'Immortal'

However, reverse walking is occasionally depicted in Chinese tales of Gods and Immortals. Some Immortals simply walk backward. Others ride their animal back to front. An exemplary figure would be Zhang Guo Lao, one of The Eight Immortals, who is often portrayed as an old man sitting on his donkey, facing backward. Reverse travelling has become a kind of trademark for certain Immortals.

Reverse walking and riding is often interpreted as an expression of appreciation toward an underlying concept. Although the walking itself is extremely powerful and potent, it is, nevertheless, still only a manifestation of that ideology.

Reversing directions and allocations offers engineers new possibilities of change. It is a method of bringing new forms of dynamics into motion. This idea is not limited to the physical arts. It is also often used in other Chinese cultural arts such as Feng Shui. Reverse breathing is another manifestation of this concept (see pages 34–41).

Walking forward feels natural, whereas walking backward contradicts your instincts and intuition. It feels as if you are walking against the wind or swimming against the current. Although immense effort is often needed to sustain reverse walking, the rewards are always substantial.

Great masters of the martial, physical, and spiritual arts have studied and practised the unique features of reverse walking. It has become an important method of training whatever your goal may be, whether it is for cultivating health, physical skill, longevity, or enlightenment.

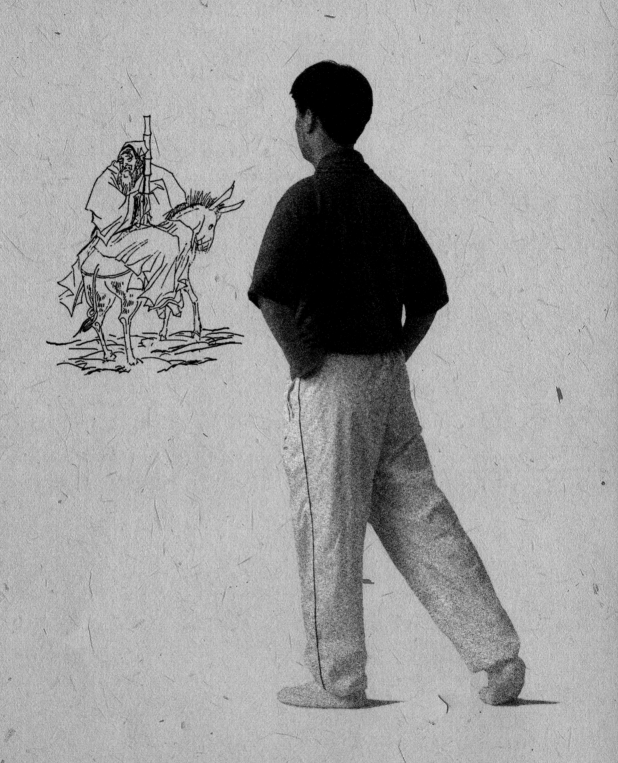

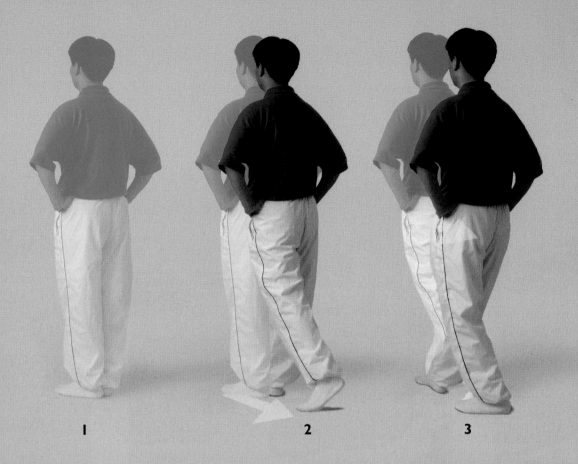

1

2

3

1 Stand comfortably straight with your heels touching. Rest both hands on your hips without tensing your shoulders. Even though you are walking backward, look forward purposefully. Do not let your gaze waver or become empty.

2 Transfer most of your weight onto the right leg without moving your centre. Gently circle your left foot backward in an arc and touch the ground behind you with your toes. Do not step too far back otherwise you will lose your balance. Avoid twisting your waist; everything above the waist should remain still.

3 Plant your left heel gently but firmly on the ground. Glide your upper body backward so that your weight is now mostly on your left leg. Avoid tilting your upper body back and sticking your bottom out. Keep everything above your waist relatively unchanged – only your centre has moved. Your upper body should remain at the same level.

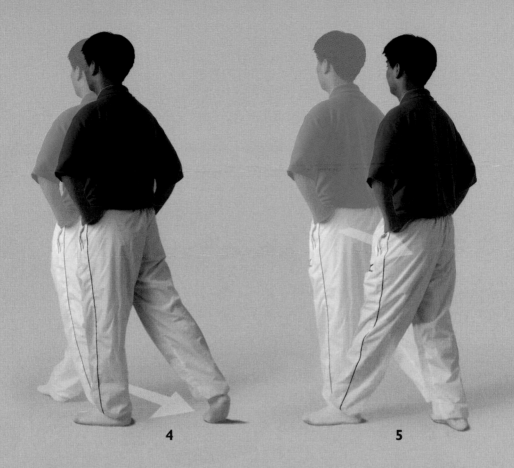

4

5

4 Circle the right foot back, slowly, and let the toes touch the floor. Your stride should be comfortably gauged to maintain balance. The leg movements should not affect your upper body. Keep your weight mostly on the left leg. Your centre is unmoved.

5 Plant your right heel firmly on the floor. Shift your weight slowly back over your right leg. Avoid turning or twisting your waist during the movement. Your right leg is now moderately bent and your left leg is almost straight. This is a mirror reflection of step 3. You should be facing the same direction throughout the sequence.

Afterwards, slowly swing your left foot back and proceed to step 2. Continue the sequence from there.

Carefree Walking of the Taoists

Taoism (pronounced Dow-ism) is one of three major schools of thought in China. It is the only native religion of Chinese people, since Confucianism cannot truly be regarded as a religion. The thoughts and ideologies of Taoism have helped shape Chinese lives for more than two thousand years. Its influence has spread to neighbouring East Asian cultures, such as Korea, Japan, and Vietnam.

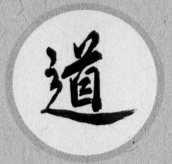

'Taoist'

Within Taoism, however, is a fundamental division that is often unheard of by the general public. On one side, we have religious Taoism, filled with Immortals, Gods, rituals, and spiritual mysteries; everything one would expect from a religion. On the other side, we have philosophical Taoism. Central to this Taoist spirit is the figure, Lao Tse, and his work, *Tao Te Ching*. This text can be translated as 'The Classic of the Way and its Power'. Lao Tse is considered to be the founder of philosophical Taoism.

Philosophical Taoism focuses on the unification of man and Heaven. These Taoists are philosophers and academics rather than priests. Their aim is to recognize and adopt an impartial existence within the universe. In this way, they seek to follow the order of Nature and disavow any selfish and deliberate actions. Particular to this school of thought is their dismissal of learned sageliness. They endeavour to embrace the simple and the primitive.

This system of walking originates from the philosophical, academic side of Taoism. In their cultivation of the mind and the spirit, these Taoists often disregarded their body. To compensate, they developed many simple but potent exercises to induce health in accordance with their doctrines. Their primary goal was mental and spiritual enhancement. This is the root of the walking exercise described here.

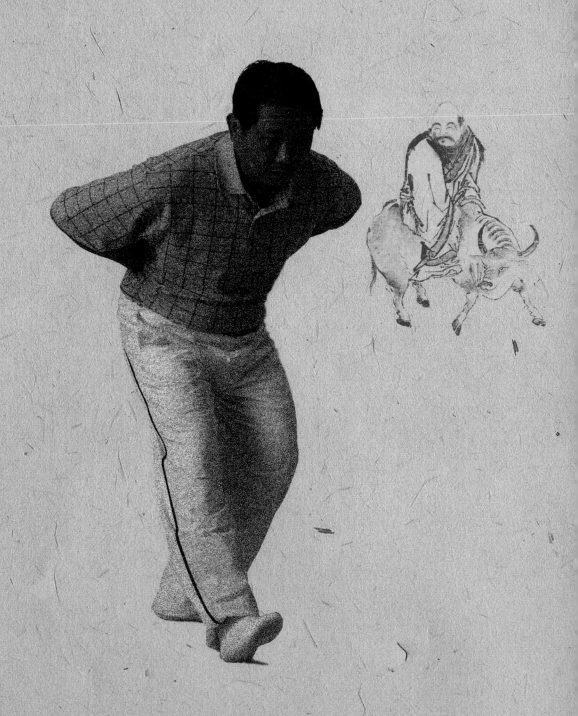

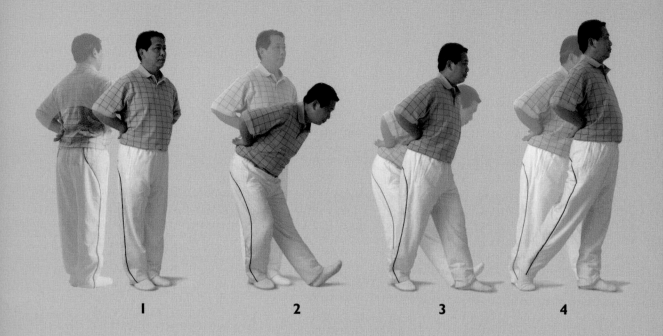

1   2   3   4

1 Stand erect with your heels together. Place your hands on your lower back, resting the backs of your hands and wrists at waist level. Try to avoid raising your elbows and shoulders.

2 Turn your body and your gaze slightly to the left. Take a step forward with your left foot, touching the ground only with the heel. Bend your right knee while keeping the left one straight. Bend forward at the waist, but avoid collapsing your chest. Keep most of your weight on the right leg.

3 Begin bringing your torso up and forward. Straighten up by pushing your belly forward. Place the rest of your left foot firmly down on the ground. The upper body should be relatively still.

4 Raise the right heel as you straighten yourself fully, transferring most of your weight onto your left leg and pushing your belly even further forward.

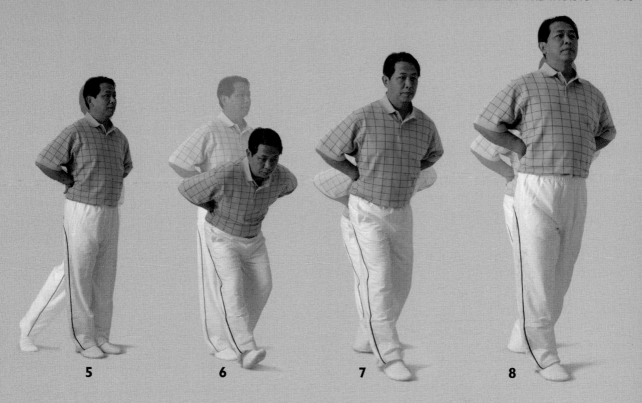

5   **6**   **7**   **8**

5 Gently bring your right foot forward to join your left, as you return to the upright posture shown in step 1.

6 Now, perform the same movements to the other side. Turn your body slightly to the right and take a step forward with your right foot. Let only your heel touch the ground. Without shifting your weight forward, bow your body moderately. Bend your left knee, but keep your right leg straight.

7 Straighten your whole body gradually by bringing your weight forward and unfolding yourself. Place the toes of your right foot down on the ground and straighten your left knee.

8 Bring your belly forward until it protrudes slightly. Lift your left heel and straighten both legs. Let your gaze rise slightly above the horizon. From here, bring your left foot to join your right, and restart the sequence from step 1.

Forward Walking of the Buddhists

It is no real surprise that some aspects of Buddhism are found here, in this chapter. After all, it is one of the four principle roots of Chi Kung. However, the relationship is actually much deeper and more intertwined with Chinese culture. Buddhism is also one of the chief origins of Chinese martial arts – more commonly known as Kung Fu – and its story is very much loved by the Chinese people.

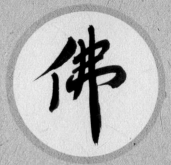

'Buddhist'

Legend says that Bodhidharma (Ta-Mo in Chinese), after attaining enlightenment, travelled to China to spread his doctrine. In his travels, he came across a Buddhist monastery in the province of Hunan. There, he sought refuge and discovered a company of resident monks with weak constitutions and failing health. Bodhidharma taught a series of health-enhancing exercises to these monks and integrated them into their existing routine. From that time on, the monks in that monastery were no longer restricted to just chanting and meditation.

With time and various inputs from other martial arts, physical and body arts flourished immeasurably within that monastery. Over a thousand years later, it became a famous establishment with a legacy of martial traditions. It is the world famous Buddhist temple of Shaolin in Central China. Despite the colourful development and legacy of Shaolin, its primary objective is still the cultivation of health.

The hand gesture of this walking system is a distinctive mark of Buddhism. Often, Buddhist monks hold this sign as a form of greeting. In Buddhism, hand gestures are an inspiring form of language and symbolism. This particular gesture, of gently clasping two hands together in front of the chest, is known as the *namaskara mudra*. It also conveys the meaning of adoration and prayer.

People often have the impression that Buddhist practice involves only sitting, meditating, and chanting. Stillness and tranquillity is, after all, the Buddhist theme. However, participation in body movement is not uncommon. Depending on the sect and the occasion, monks may walk and chant together. The routine of walking is a real part of Buddhist practice.

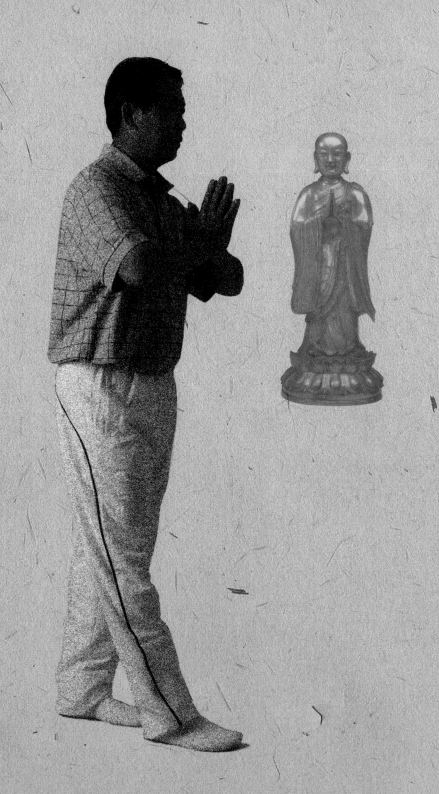

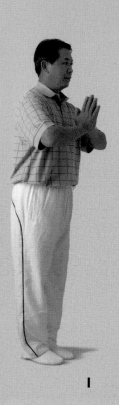

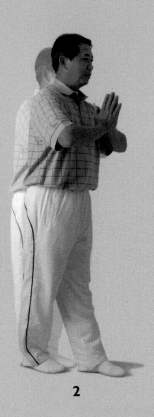

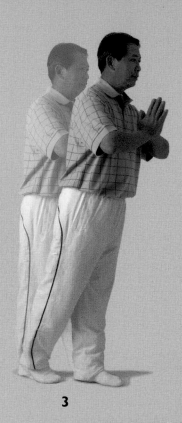

1

2

3

1 Stand upright and gaze forward. Let your heels touch, but have a slight gap between the front of the feet. Raise your hands in front of your chest and let them clap softly together. The palms and the fingers should be in full contact. Avoid lifting your elbows or your shoulders too high.

2 Take a small step forward with your left foot, but keep both legs straight. There should be no change whatsoever above the waist. Avoid moving your centre, and keep most of your weight on your right leg.

3 Shift your body forward so that most of your weight is on your left leg. Your right heel is slightly raised, but the leg remains straight. Tilt your body forward slightly. Try not to bend your upper body or collapse your chest. Everything above your waist should be relatively still.

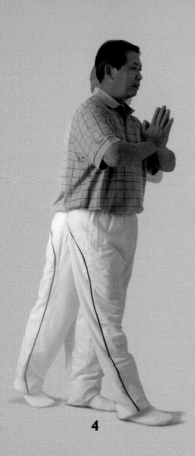

4

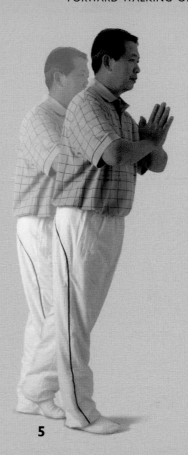

5

4 Without making any other movements, bring your right foot to the front. Make sure you are well balanced on your left leg. Your upper body should remain slightly tilted.

5 Bring your weight forward, toward the right leg. Keep both legs straight at all times. Lift your left heel so that only the front of your foot touches the ground. From there, step forward with your left foot and continue the sequence.

Stationary Walking of the Medics

Chinese traditional medicine is the biggest alternative to modern medicine. It is practised across the world, and is probably the longest continuing practice of medicine in world history. The expertise of Chinese medicine is not limited to curing sickness and healing wounds. It is also dedicated to the improvement of general health, and to the cultivation of longevity. In other words, Chinese medicine is also a form of preventive health care.

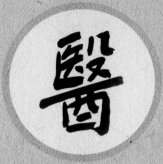

'Medic(al)'

In Chinese physiology, the human body contains a number of channels through which human energy flows. They extend to the tip of each finger and thumb. The heels and the toes are also linked to various channels.

Unlike spiritual or internal body arts, Chinese medicinal exercises place greater emphasis on movement than stillness. This walking system stimulates and encourages human Chi so that it flows with greater strength and vitality. The hands, feet, and waist are all in a motion that has been intricately composed by past Chinese doctors.

Walking is a great way of executing such medicinal body motion. It is familiar to people of all ages. Most people walk on a daily basis. The system here is an example of stationary walking. Steps are taken but you are not travelling anywhere. Stationary walking may appear strange, but it is actually very practical. First of all, it is space-efficient and can, therefore, be practised almost anywhere. There is no change of direction. It is also suitable for the elderly and people with minor mobility problems.

In some ways, Chinese medicine favours stationary walking, because it is relatively safe. Being stationary, you can more conveniently be in the company of others. A support, such as a chair, can be readily at hand. The chances of tripping are also significantly reduced since your feet are not raised from the ground. As well as the internal energy workout, these medical considerations are also incorporated into this walking system.

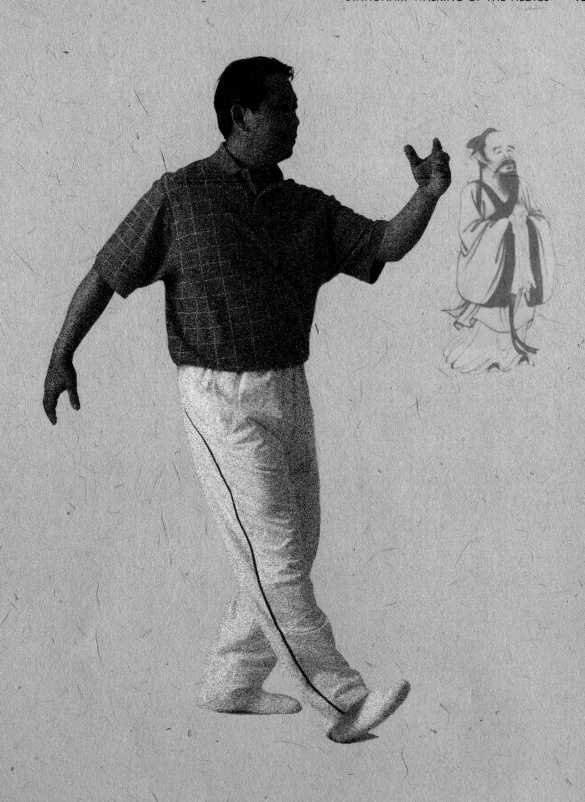

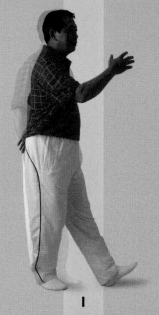

1

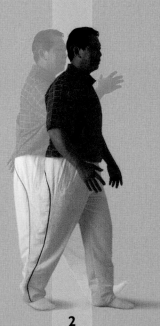

2

1 Stand straight and let your heels touch. Allow your arms to hang naturally from your shoulders. Breathe gently and deeply until you are calm and ready to begin.

Take a step forward with your left foot. Your heel is on the ground, but the front of the foot is raised. Turn your body minutely to the left and raise your right arm in front of you – breathe in as you do so. The right hand faces the left. Your left hand sways back a little. Your weight is mostly upon your right leg.

2 Gently and slowly swing your left arm forward and your right arm down. At the same time, place your left foot down flat on the ground. Breathe out slowly and evenly.

3 Swing the left arm up until your hand is at head-level. Your right arm swings back past your side. Turn your body and gaze to the right. Shift your weight forward, raising your right heel.

4 Swing your arms again, this time, your left arm down and your right arm up. Breathe in again slowly as you do this. Plant your right heel down and return your weight back to the right leg.

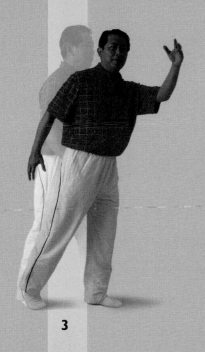

3

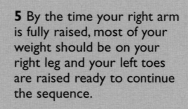

5 By the time your right arm is fully raised, most of your weight should be on your right leg and your left toes are raised ready to continue the sequence.

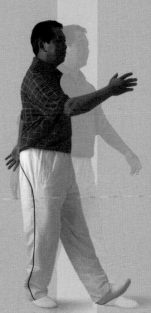

5

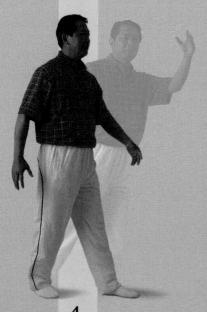

4

Variation *The sequence shown is for men. For women, the variation in the walking system is a mirror reflection.*

From the standing posture where both heels touch, step forward with the right foot. The right toes do not meet the ground. The left arm is raised in front of you, and the right hand swings backward. Breathe in as you move your arms.

Swap the role of both arms by swinging the right arm forward and the left hand back. Lower the front of your right foot. At the same time, exhale slowly and evenly.

Swing your right arm until your right hand is high in front of you. Remember to lift your left heel.

Xing Yi Walking of the Martial Artists

This walking system is named after a particular school of Chinese martial art. However, its roots go even deeper and further back into history.

During an age when wars were not uncommon in China, military developments were thriving. Long weapons, such as spears, were often employed, and soldiers proficient in wielding such weapons were formed into special units. These weapons were often uncomfortably long and heavy. Those that carried them marched forward, packed tightly together as one unified force. Their combat techniques may have been limited but, collectively, they were unstoppable.

Among the less accountable histories, General Yueh Fei of the Sung Dynasty is said to have developed a martial discipline for his soldiers. This army became a prominent and powerful force in the history of China. Their discipline was rumoured to be a founding stone of what later evolved into the martial school of Xing Yi.

Somewhere and somehow during the course of Chinese history, martial and physical artists noticed this military training, particularly the long weapons training; the powerful forward exertion of strength; the simple yet extremely potent movements; and the efficiency of body control. All of these skills were of great interest to the martial artists.

In transition, the underlying essences of the military movements were distilled and developed. The steps, the power exertions, and the power allocations were refined, and philosophy, breathing methodology, and Chinese internal physiology were introduced. These changes transformed a substance of the military into a substance of martial art. It became a new system of walking in its own right and is now one of the core practices in Chinese soft martial arts.

This walking exercise – though a distant offspring of military training – can also be practised for the cultivation of longevity and health. Although your centre still needs to sink slightly, the overall sensation is lighter and more levitated. The walking sequence illustrated here is practised mainly for its health benefits.

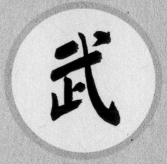

'Martial'

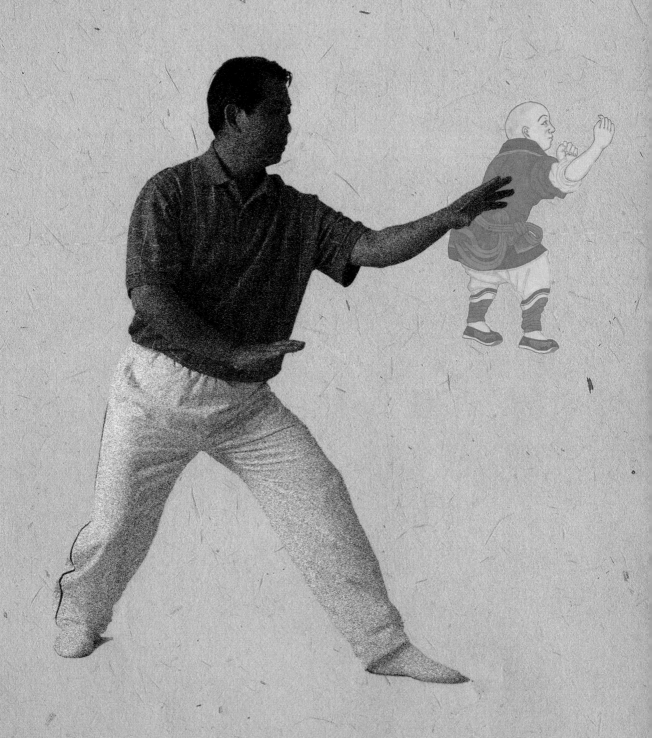

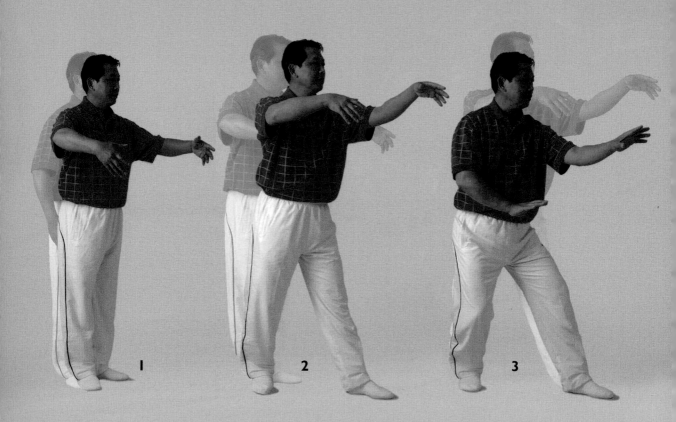

1   2   3

1 Stand erect with your arms hanging gently by your sides. Keep your heels together. The front of your feet separate and at a slight angle. Gaze forward, breathing calmly. Slowly bring your arms up by circling them from the sides. Your left arm is further away from your body than your right arm. In other words, your right elbow is more bent than your left. At the same time, turn your body slightly to the right.

2 When your hands are about level with your shoulders, bring your left foot forward. Turn your arms so that the palms face down, keeping your wrists loose and gentle. Try to avoid lifting and tensing your shoulders.

3 Sink your weight down and bend your knees. Lower your left elbow until the hand is at approximately shoulder-level. Lower your right arm until the hand is level with your belly. You should now have 60 per cent of your weight on the right leg and 40 per cent on the left. Keep your upper body upright.

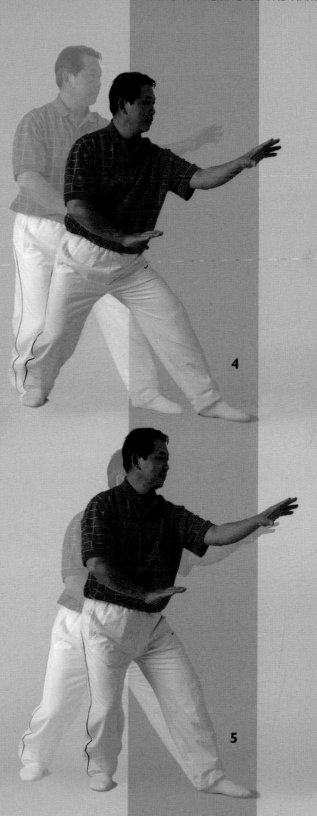

4 Step forward again with your left foot. At the same time, shift and tilt your upper body minutely forward in a slow but powerful gesture. Keep your gaze straight ahead at all times.

5 Bring your right foot forward without changing the direction of the foot. Your upper body returns to the upright posture of step 3. Continue the sequence in a loop from here, repeating steps 3 to 5 as you very slowly proceed forward.

Balance Walking of the Boatmen

China is a geographical treasure house. Its landscapes vary from deserts to marshlands, plains to valleys. Local customs and cultures vary across the country in harmony with their local environment.

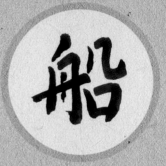

'Boat'

In the midlands of China dwells a culture of water. The central region of the country is full of rivers and lakes. Many cities are built next to, or even on the water, much like Venice. These places have brought forth many customs and traditions. It was from this culture of swimming, sailing, fishing, and ferrying that the inspiration for this walking system evolved and took life.

The life of a fisherman or a ferryman can be rather harsh and demanding. To compensate, a healthy lifestyle and routine are crucial. Their lives can be completely intertwined with their boats. Many boatmen literally live and raise their families on boats, and this way of life has created a unique set of circumstances.

The tranquillity of the sea, rivers, and lakes offers them ideal conditions for natural meditation. The constant association with nature and wildlife brings a deep understanding and philosophy. The various intricate daily tasks performed on a boat or ship give them an appreciation of dynamic movement and mechanisms. The continuous rocking of the boat teaches them balance. The long waits for a catch or a fare develop the virtue of patience, and offer them opportunities for training. Under these various complementing circumstances, this walking system came into existence.

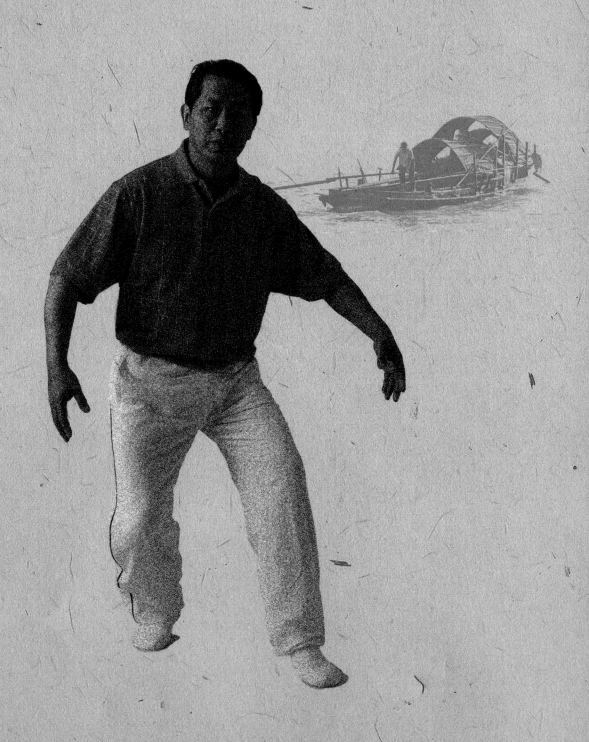

Please note *As this walk is freestyle, we are unable to number the steps for you.*

Stand upright with your heels together and your feet 45 degrees apart. Let your arms hang naturally, palms facing in. Allow a fairly large space between your arms and your sides. Your fingers should be apart and naturally straight.

Step forward and start to walk randomly. Imagine you are standing on the deck of a boat that is swaying left and right, to and fro. The current is strong but not ferocious.

Begin walking in a manner befitting a seasoned boatman. Familiarize yourself with the rhythm of the waves and the rocking of the deck. Walk not with the aim of going somewhere; walk just in order to harmonize with the rhythm. Move and bend so that your balance continually realigns.

You can step forward or to the side; occasionally, you may even step backward. All these directions are at your disposal. But, choose your directions wisely. Overall, this walk may appear disorderly and chaotic, with no system or structure. However, this is far from true. The orderliness is within.

When taking a step, your feet can be close together or moderately apart. Never take too big a step, or straighten your legs completely. Keeping the knees bent at all times is key to maintaining balance. A true boatman understands his own centre and plays with his balance like a toy.

Let your arms sway a little with the rhythm of the waves. Use them as balancing tools that move instinctively to assist your centre. Your arms should sway as if they are weightless and somehow breathing.

Everything is in a state of flux, and depends only on the moment. You may sink your weight low or lift it high. Your centre is in perpetual motion. Your weight does not rest evenly on both legs; it gently oscillates between the two.

Make use of the full flexibility of your feet. Raise and lower your heels and the front of the feet independently, to maintain your balance.

Let your mind direct the rocking of the imaginary deck in a gentle, rhythmic pace. You need not walk with any particular haste. Let everything be instinctive and instantaneous, with no imposed pattern of movement. Do not allow yourself to become wild and erratic; remember to stay relaxed and focused on your centre and your balance.

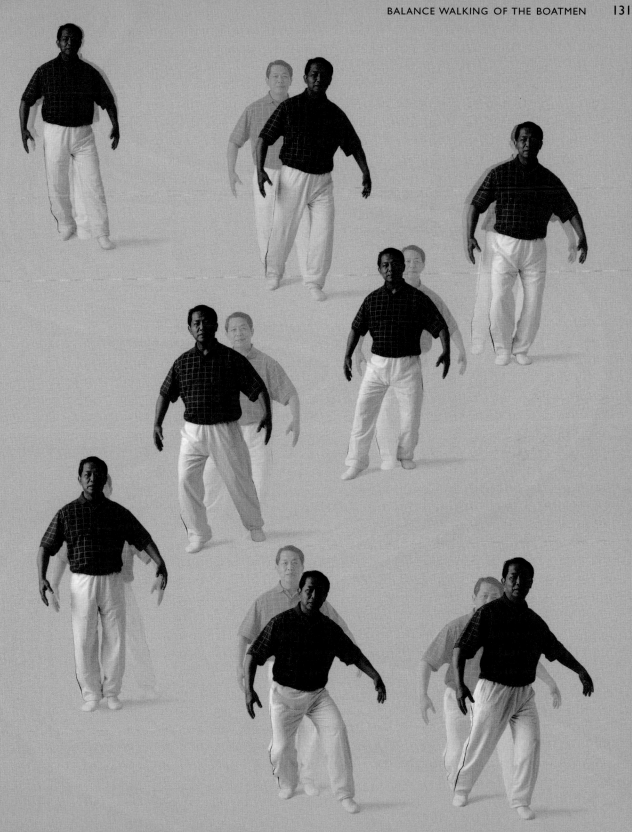

March Walking of the Military

The name for this particular walking system is drawn from the fact that its simple appearance bears some resemblance to the marching of soldiers. Like many terms in Chinese martial arts, its name is chosen to enable you to more readily remember the movements.

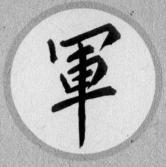

'Military'

Even during those times in ancient China when the crafts of war were flourishing, marching was unheard of in the military. Systems of step walking for engagements and battle formations were plentiful and well studied, but there were few records in existence of a walking style designed for the sole purpose of unified mobility.

The emphasis of this walking system is on its simplicity. Like the Wu Chi posture – which is meant to be the foremost and most natural of standing postures for a human body – this walk is intended to be the primal system of steps.

Its apparent plainness and stressed simplicity is the key to its potency. However, do not think that the internal working of energy in this walking system is equally plain and simple. Simply because the name and appearance are closely associated, do not fall into the trap of confusing and merging this walking system with contemporary military marches. There is a vast difference between their underlying essences, which sets them a world apart.

The purpose of a military march is to display collective strength and bring numerous individuals to a single rhythm. The essence here is to stimulate your Chi circulation with pressures, motions, and alignments of the body.

Do not allow your pace to quicken just because this exercise seems effortless. Let the rhythm of your steps be gentle and natural. This particular walking system is my own contribution after decades of experience and understanding.

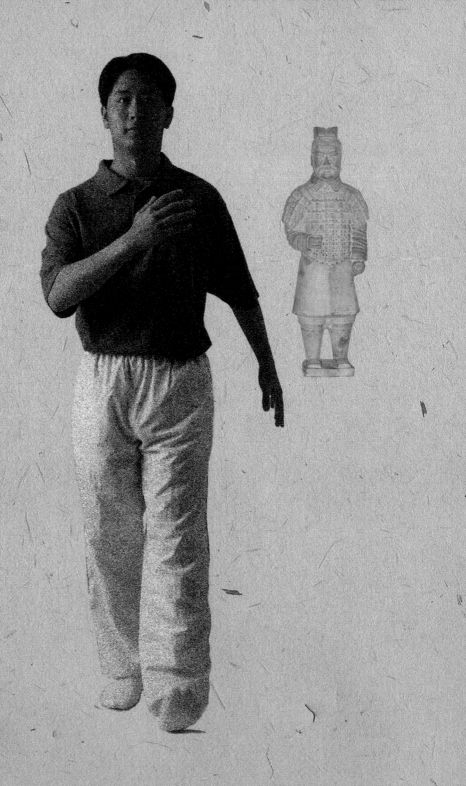

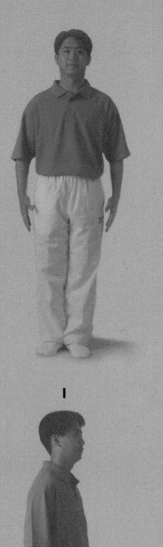

1

1 Stand upright, facing forward. Let your heels touch, but have your feet apart at approximately 45 degrees. Allow your arms to hang comfortably by your sides, palms facing inward. Have your fingers slightly apart and naturally curved. Loosen your shoulders, elbows, and knees. Despite the name of this system, do not stand in a stiff and tense military manner. Breathe through your nose, calmly and deeply.

2 Take a step forward with your left foot. Your intention is to avoid bending your knees – both legs should remain naturally straight. At the same time, raise your right hand in front of your chest over the vertical centre of your body, and swing your left hand back, elbow slightly bent. Don't bring your right arm too close to your body.

Keep your wrists, elbows, and shoulders relaxed. The step should not be so large that the straight alignment of your legs is broken. Rest your left heel on the ground.

Avoid moving your centre, and keep most of your weight on your right leg.

Variation *You can perform this walking system in a discontinuous manner. After taking each step, pause for one or two seconds before moving again.*

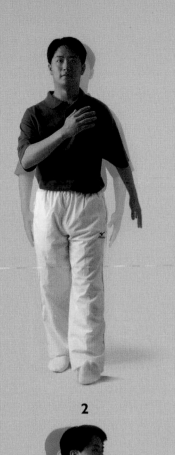

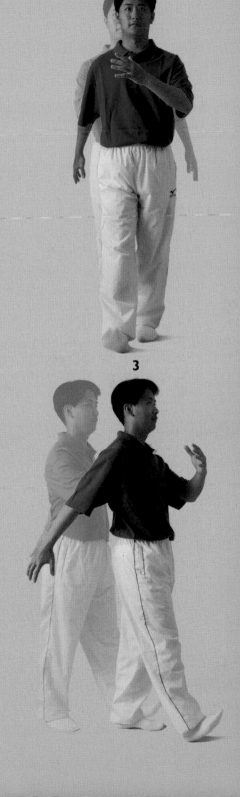

3 Allow the rest of your left foot to gradually touch the ground. Let it press down with gentle firmness. Allow the pressure against the sole of your foot to work to your advantage as you bring the right foot forward to rest on its heel. As you do this, swing the left hand forward and the right hand back.

Continue the march, stepping forward with your left foot and swinging your right hand forward. Remember, your right hand swings up to chest level and passes the centre line of your body, as shown in step 2. Try not to move your centre line laterally.

2

3

Circular Walking of Da Cheng Chuan

This final walking system is rather demanding in terms of bearing and spatial coordination. The direction is circular; therefore, your linear alignment is constantly changing.

This particular system of circular walking was devised by Grand Master Wang Xiang Zhai. He drew inspiration from, among other things, a system known as Pa Kua steps. That walking system outlines an octagon in which the practitioner moves and turns in accordance to the eight directions. The emphasis of Pa Kua steps is on straight lines and careful crossing of the legs. This system takes on a smoother shape. Here, instead of a polygon, we have a circle. Instead of straight lines, the feet move in curves. Grand Master Wang Xiang Zhai developed this walking system with a different emphasis, and with a different purpose in mind.

This step sequence is a crystallization of three special features. First, the line of each step draws an arc. This is known as 'the curve step'. Second, the foot slides along the surface of the ground as if it is surfing on mud. These steps are known as 'wading-on-mud'. Third, the foot movements take on a pattern known in Taoism as 'the seven stars steps'. Grand Master Wang Xiang Zhai's walking system is an artistic and practical unification of these three features.

This exercise not only trains your mental and physical coordination, it also helps develop your directional flexibility. The size of the circle you will be marking is quite flexible. It simply depends on the availability of space. If necessary, you can mark a small circle for space efficiency. You may also choose to place an object at the centre of the circle to assist you in your orientation.

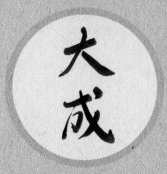

'Da Cheng (Great Accomplishment)'

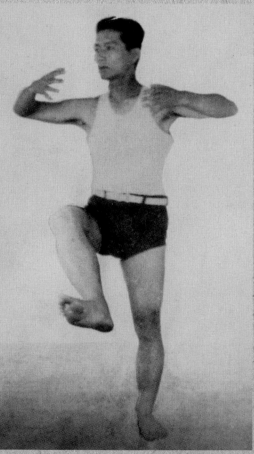

Right *Professor Yu as a young man, practises a more energetic form of circular walking.*

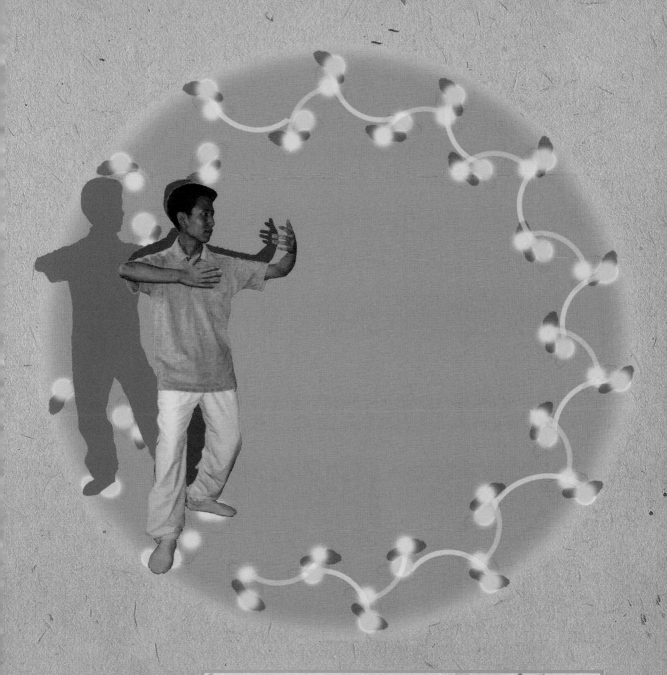

Please note As you perform the steps, keep the moving foot parallel to, and as close to the floor as possible.

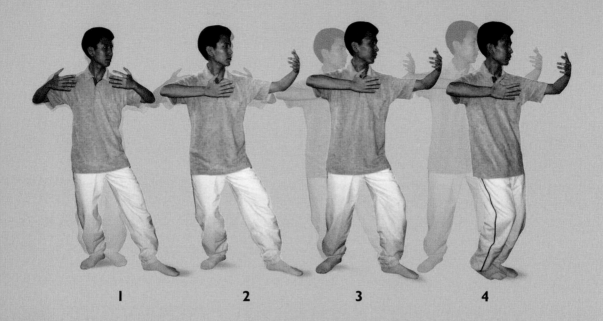

1   2   3   4

Please note *In this exercise you are marking a circle in a counterclockwise direction.*

Stand upright with your heels together. Gaze forward and relax, letting your arms hang loosely at your sides.

Bring both arms up slowly as you bend your knees. Your palms face your shoulders, and your fingers are apart and softly curved.

1 Turn your head to the left and transfer most of your weight to your right leg. Step with your left foot out to the left. Avoid moving your body or your centre.

2 Turn your body slightly to the left. Move your left hand out further away from you by unfolding the elbow slightly. The right hand moves inward toward the centre line of your chest.

3 Shift your centre towards the left leg. Avoid tilting your body forward or leaning back. Everything above the waist should remain relatively still.

4 As you balance yourself on the left leg, bring the right foot up so that your feet once again touch each other. However, your right foot rests on the ground with only the toes (see page 137). Notice that both knees are bent, but in different ways.

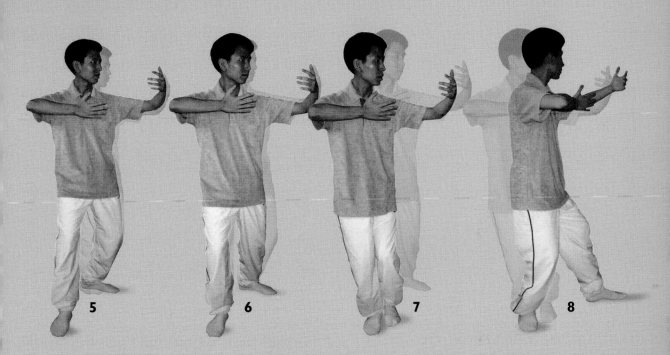

5

6

7

8

5 Keeping your weight mostly in the left leg, step out with your right foot to your right.

6 Without changing the direction of your gaze and your body, shift your weight forward onto your right leg.

7 Bring your left foot forward to rest beside your right foot. Keep your left heel elevated as you do this.

8 Turn your gaze and your body to the left and step the left foot out in an arc in that direction. Your head, arms, and body should be relatively still. The degree you turn is dependent on how large a circle you are marking. Except for the difference in direction, this is now the same posture as in step 5. Repeat the sequence from there until you have drawn a full circle.

Final words

In this book, you have come across a variety of steps and walking systems. Some of these are straightforward, while some are lengthy. Some are very simple and some extremely complicated. To many of you, this will have been a journey of discovery. To others, a long voyage of study and education. Try not to be overwhelmed or discouraged by the vast and colourful spectrum of this art. All things, great or small, must begin somewhere.

It does not matter if you are young or in your prime. A farmer always prepares for the coming winter. This is an ancient but valid piece of wisdom. It is always easier to preserve and promote better health when you are well. When you are sick, it is much more difficult and time-consuming. Sometimes, it can be too late.

Preservation of health is always preferable to the restoration of health. It is unwise to think that because you are young and strong now, you do not need to prepare for the any future decline of your health.

CHOOSING THE RIGHT STEPS

The art of walking can be a huge labyrinth in which you may sometimes feel lost. You want someone to tell you which is the most suitable step system for you. With time and patience, you will find the right steps for yourself. The best way to walk is to do so naturally. Allow your body to tell you which steps are right for you. Your role is to learn to listen carefully.

However, it is not wise to dwell too much on this search. Like hunting, sometimes, the more you chase your prey, the faster it runs away. There is an old Chinese fable that parents teach their children. It was meant to be an analogy, bearing a metaphoric interpretation. However, for us, it is conveniently quite literal.

This comical story from the ancient Chinese philosopher, Zhuang Tzu, teaches the lesson that you must not be overwhelmed by the vast variety of walking systems out there and neglect your own natural walking style.

WALKING STEPS

As the Chinese language is pictographic, many words and concepts are expressed by two or more symbols, allowing the reader to interpret abstract meanings that cannot be expressed with just one symbol. Not all abstract ideas are graphically represented, sometimes there is a phonetic ingredient, but many of these no longer provide clues to pronunciation.

'Walking' and 'steps' share the same character, originally represented as two feet in succession, indicating that a person is walking forward or has taken a step. This image evolved through time as we see in these copies.

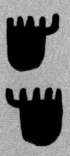

EARLIEST SYMBOL
When Chinese writing was still purely pictographic, the abstract concept of 'walking' was expressed with the left foot in front of the right.

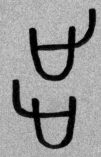

ORACLE BONE SCRIPT (Jia Gu Wen)
The two foot images appear to have simplified, illustrating mainly the big toes. Some lesser toes are eliminated, and the soles are not filled.

LEARNING STEPS AT HAN DAN

There was once a young man who lived in the countryside, and who walked in a very awkward manner. Because of this he often tripped and fell. One day he came across someone who told him of the great city of Han Dan, where the people walked properly and elegantly. The young man was advised to stay at that city for some time in order to learn to walk correctly.

The young man heeded this counsel and went to live in Han Dan. There he saw people walking in all manners and styles. He studied carefully, and started to imitate each one.

Time passed and the people of his home-town awaited his return. Eventually, the young man came home but, to the astonishment of everyone, he returned crawling on the ground. The young man had become so confused and overwhelmed that he had forgotten how to walk at all!

WALKING TIPS

The accumulated time we spend walking in our life time is immense. If we could harness these walking moments to greater efficiency, the rewards could be profound.

Plan your time more generously. Avoid a schedule that is too tight. Do not make yourself walk in a hurry. You should enjoy the pleasure of walking. Take your steps at a natural and comfortable pace. Breathe at a relaxing rhythm as you walk.

If your schedule is free, take some time to walk after every meal. If outside is cold, wet, or unsafe, simply walk around the room.

This may feel troublesome to some people at first but, in time, you will learn to appreciate the simplicity of walking and the pleasure it offers.

For the ladies, sinking your weight to the front of your feet when you walk will help improve the curvature of your calves. By bringing the weight to the heels, you are improving the lines of the thighs as you walk.

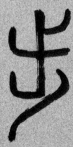

BRONZE SCRIPT (Jin Wen)
The top graphic component remains unchanged, while the lower component is slightly modified.

LESSER SEAL SCRIPT (Xiao Zhuan)
Here, the character undergoes a relatively major transformation. However, there are still some resemblances to the foot images given enough imagination.

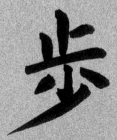

STANDARD SCRIPT (Kai Shu)
This is the 'walking' character in use today in both the 'Traditional' and the 'Simplified' scripts.

Index

ABOUT THE AUTHOR

Master Lam Kamchuen has devoted his life to the classical arts of Chinese culture. He has brought these to the West and introduced the unique practices of Chinese health care to millions through his books and videos.

Born in Hong Kong, Master Lam began his formal instruction in the martial arts at the age of eleven. Studying under masters such as Lung Tse Chung and Yim Sheung Mo, he was trained in Choy Lee Fut, Northern Shaolin Kung Fu, Iron Palm, and Tai Chi Chuan.

He became a disciple of Professor Yu Yong Nian, the world's leading authority on Zhan Zhuang, the most powerful of all forms of Chi Kung – and is now a recognized lineage holder in that tradition.

Master Lam came to the West in 1975 and has developed a wide following of students throughout the United Kingdom and Europe. He is the author of a dozen books including his ground-breaking Chi Kung trilogy: *The Way of Energy*, *The Way of Healing*, and *The Way of Power*.

The Lam Association, established by Master Lam, is devoted to preserving and teaching the classical arts that promote health and wellbeing. You may contact the association as follows:

The Lam Association
1 Hercules Road
London, SE1 7DP
Tel/Fax: 0044 (0)20 7261 9049
Mobile: 0044 (0)7831 802598
Website: www.lamassociation.org

AUTHOR'S ACKNOWLEDGEMENT

For the opportunity to have become who I am and be where I am, I must first offer thanks to the masters of all the arts which I have learned. They have been very patient, and were like fathers to me. I owe to them my knowledge and understanding of these arts. I must also give thanks to all the past masters across the ages that have preserved and contributed to the arts presented in this book.

To my family, I owe much gratitude. Their continuing patience and support are an important factor in my achievements. My wife, Kaisin, has helped me over the years in every way, so that I am freely able to concentrate on these arts. I am grateful to my sons for their willingness to continue these traditions and arts. On this occasion, I would like to thank Tinhun, my youngest son, who took time to pose as a model

in this book. Tinyu, my middle son, has also helped me greatly with the text for this book.

A word of appreciation to Bridget Morley, the designer. We have worked together on many occasions and despite the elevating demands I place on her, she still continues to exceed my expectations.

Last, but not least, I give many special thanks and gratitude to people who make this book a reality. This is my first business association with Alison Goff, the chief executive officer of Octopus Publishing Group, and she has been warm and welcoming. Patrick Nugent has guided the direction of this book as he has done with my past works. Cindy Engel kindly edited the final text, and Paul Forrester performed the photography. A special round of thanks also to the many people who work backstage.

IMAGE CREDITS All calligraphy by Master Lam. Studio photography of Master Lam and Tinhun Lam by Paul Forrester. Photographs supplied by Getty Images: 26 Richard H Johnston, 63 Christian Michaels, 73 Gandee Vasan. Remaining images supplied by Master Lam. Collage/image manipulation by Bridget Morley.